I'm Thought*ing*

On **ADHD**, **Dyslexia**, and **Parenting Outside the Box**

PH ACHARYA

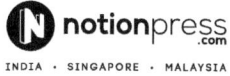

INDIA · SINGAPORE · MALAYSIA

Notion Press

Old No. 38, New No. 6
McNichols Road, Chetpet
Chennai - 600 031

First Published by Notion Press 2020
Copyright © PH Acharya 2020
All Rights Reserved.

ISBN 978-1-64850-603-1

This book has been published with all efforts taken to make the material error-free after the consent of the author. However, the author and the publisher do not assume and hereby disclaim any liability to any party for any loss, damage, or disruption caused by errors or omissions, whether such errors or omissions result from negligence, accident, or any other cause.

While every effort has been made to avoid any mistake or omission, this publication is being sold on the condition and understanding that neither the author nor the publishers or printers would be liable in any manner to any person by reason of any mistake or omission in this publication or for any action taken or omitted to be taken or advice rendered or accepted on the basis of this work. For any defect in printing or binding the publishers will be liable only to replace the defective copy by another copy of this work then available.

Contents

About the Author, Editor 5
Preface: A Disclaimer 11
Acknowledgements 13
Foreword 15

1. And Then I Begun to Do Like This… 19
2. Pappa, I Was Very in Tension…. 27
3. Mumma Doesn't Know Anything Only! 33
4. Do You Memember? 45
5. But Morely, I Want to Do That... 55
6. No Fault of Kārtikéya's 65
7. Little a Bit Medicine 73
8. Don't Undera… underamamestimate Me! 81
9. When I Grow Up, My Height Will Be Big! 87
10. Did He Went from School? 97

Et Tu? 109
Expert-Speak 121
Epilogue 129

About the Author, Editor

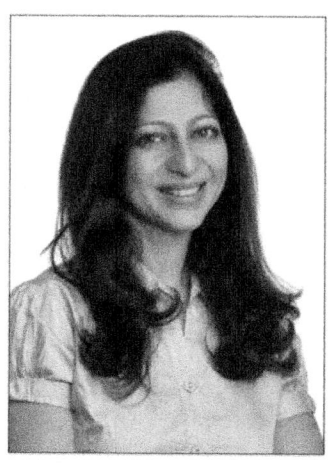

PH Acharya is a Life Coach and Graphotherapist. She is an Associate Certified Coach (ACC-accredited) who also has Marshall Goldsmith's stamp of approval, making her one amongst the most sought-after group of corporate and life coaches in the industry.

Based in Mumbai, she works with individuals and multinational companies alike. She has worked as a mentor with the *Self-Employed Women's Association* (SEWA), tasked with improving female entrepreneurs' efficiency and spirit. Acharya also works as a

About the Author, Editor

motivational speaker with *Sanjeevani*, which handholds underprivileged cancer patients from their diagnosis, through the process of treatment, and beyond.

This is her third book. She is the author of *Tat Tvam Asi*[1] – a collection of short stories. Her booklet *Bald is Beautiful*[2] is a chemo-patient's guide to hope and strength, and is distributed for free all over the world. As an audio-book, it has been a pillar to hundreds of patients during their treatment journey and has received an overwhelmingly positive response from their families and doctors as well.

As of 2019, Acharya lives in Mumbai with her husband and children, whom you will meet in this book. She continues to work with social-sector initiatives, which she enjoys blogging about on her LinkedIn page.

A. Ashni is the pen to Acharya's thoughts. Currently bound as her mother's marketing manager, she is a noble philanthropist who gives away this labour for free. Since 2017, Ashni has worked on all of Acharya's projects, including *Tat Tvam Asi*, and has the stellar record of never once complaining to HR.

Ashni was bribed into editing this book with the promise of a pet[3]. She requests that the audience forgive any errors and accredit all oversight to her frustration

---

[1] Available on Amazon.in.

[2] Displaying and distributing at clinics, hospitals, support-groups, and other spaces where patients benefit. Contact pinkyhacharya@gmail.com for free copies for your establishment.

[3] ...or threatened with the promise to *never* adopt a pet. It's a matter of perspective.

upon being emotionally blackmailed (yet again) into soul-sucking labour.

She never got that pet.

To Kitu.

"Don't give didi to write my book!"[4]

– Krishnav Acharya

---

[4] Krishnav has graced the English language with some grammatical gems over the last 17 years. Please enjoy...

Preface: A Disclaimer

This is our story.

At the very onset, I'd like to remind the reader that this book is not a scientific How-To on raising children with learning disabilities. My experiences are not universal; they need not be your's.

This is not a prescription. I am no degree-holding expert myself – just a mother with her experiences.

I'm Thoughting is my attempt to put forth a single testimony on what it's like to raise a child with Specific Learning Disabilities (SLDs). Parenting is a precarious game and no one has the rule book! Through trial and error, we somehow manage to bring in the new generation – sometimes thriving, sometimes scarred, and quite often both. Trying to figure out how and how much to parent is a boundless experiment. Experimenting with my son... well, let's just say I felt like a mad scientist.

How do you maintain your balance?

How do you exercise good judgement in a moment of immediacy?

How do you make peace with failing time-bound improvements?

Preface: A Disclaimer

How do you keep up the moments of genius effective parenting?

How do you catch a cloud and pin it down?

I don't know. But I can tell you what I did when faced with these questions.

I had not intended to write a book about him when he was born. So my memories with Krishnav – as memories usually go – are at times hazy. I have done my best to reconstruct every anecdote with utmost accuracy and authenticity.

With these threads I've collected from the far corners of my brain, I've tried to knit a little gift for the reader. A shawl, of sorts, you could say. Disabilities are...well, disabling. The confines society defines for PWDs (persons with disabilities) make it seem as though their fates are sealed. But disabilities lie on a spectrum of dashed lines – mobility and improvement is not impossible. I'd like to think of this shawl as a light something to wrap around when times get tough. It won't take away the cold, no. But it's something to remind you that warm mornings do come around.

So in the name of warm mornings...

Acknowledgements

"Thanking you!"

First and foremost, I thank the Almighty for this adventure. Your blessings fill me with immense hope. Gratitude for being by my family through the rougher terrains. Thank you for the faith that allows me to propel forward, knowing You're standing right behind to catch me should I stumble.

A big thank you to all those who've been instrumental in Krishnav's academic journey. Baiju and Nipan, you are his guardian angels, going the extra mile to help Krishnav actualise his passion. Words fail to express our gratitude for your unstinting support and selfless love. Your drive to look for newer pastures for him to explore was instrumental in opening doors to the road less travelled.

Thank you Manoj Sir, Manjit Sir and Kalpana Mam for holding and elevating our boy when he needed it the most.

Thank you Ashni, for being Krishnav's mentor, confidant, bodyguard, and Google. Your woke perspectives

Acknowledgements

and sensitivity help us evolve. You are the voice, the resource, the soul of this book.

Thank you Himsi, for always having my back through all my crazy ventures and for the belief that I can do it.

A most special thank you to Maharashtra Dyslexia Association (MDA), Ms. Kate Currawalla, Ms. Masarrat Khan, Ms. Afshaan Jabeen, and Ms. Rukshan Vakil for their precious time, expert suggestions, and faith in this book. A thank you also to Nayi Disha Resource Centre for their mammoth fund of knowledge.

It would be remiss not to extend my thanks and love to Jarul and Indira Thakur, Aditi and Dr. and Dr. Gandhi, and Dr. Sandeep P. T. for sharing their stories with us. Your perspectives have made this book all the richer.

Foreword

The journey of a thousand miles starts with a single step. But if you falter time and again at the first steps, disappointment and demotivation accompany you for what becomes a most frustrating journey.

In my 20+ years of experience, this rings dead true for parents of children with learning difficulties.

I've watched India's SLD landscape transform over the past 20 years. While I *can* testify that acceptance of children with disabilities is higher today, I would be lying if I said it was sufficient. Indian parents have yet not come to terms with SLDs in our children enough to warrant a pat on our collective backs.

The biggest card stacked against students is that SLDs are invisible handicaps. There are no necessarily obvious physical deformities, speech impediments, or mental / emotional disturbances that manifest visibly. Since their disability isn't visible to a stranger, those who do not know of their situation label such students as "naughty" or deliberately "mischievous".

But being labelled by others is a Tier2 problem. SLD perception in the family itself is most important. Since SLDs aren't visible, many parents / primary caregivers themselves have a hard time absorbing that their child has special needs. When a formal diagnosis or psycho-educational assessment is suggested, I've found that most parents' reaction is ye old denial. Their child is so bright! It seems ludicrous to suggest they could have a disorder / disability!

What we don't say enough is that delayed acceptance leads to delayed improvement.

Moreover, school administrators and class teachers (by and large) are not even sensitized to the *existence* of learning disabilities[5], let alone trained in SLD management in the classroom. They may (unintentionally or otherwise) subject the child to daily verbal and non-verbal shaming – comparing them with their peers, ridiculing them for their handwriting or "simple" mistakes.

This can leave indelible scars on your child's self-esteem and psyche. No wonder weak management of a learning disability today is known to lead to emotional disturbances tomorrow.

A good place for schools to start? Make teachers and parents aware of the academic assistance children may need. Boards give concessions and classroom accommodations that schools and parents may not make use of due to lack of awareness. And thus, thousands of

---

[5] Corroborated by Maharashtra Dyslexia Association (MDA). Outreach to schools is the most difficult part of working in the SLD space because more schools than you would imagine entirely deny or dismiss the existence of SLDs. [From conversations with Masarrat Khan, CEO MDA.]

children who could've had access to help are deprived of much-needed support – support that was initiated with the very intention to accomodate special needs children in mainstream education.

This book is a commendable step towards public awareness in India. PH Acharya has shared with the reader her pain, frustration, hopes, and triumphs. As unique as each parenting journey, I'm sure the reader will find comfort and healing in seeing themselves in these pages.

So dear Parent, here is your community. Enjoy!

Afshan Jabeen
Ripples Centre for Enhanced Learning
RCI Clinical Psychologist, SIS Dyslexia Therapist

Chapter One

And Then I Begun to Do Like This...

This is the story of an adventure our family never thought we'd share.

In 2002, my life was bliss. I had my soulmate, Himanshu, on one arm and my four year-old genius, Ashni, on the other. We were your typical Gujarati Mumbaikar upper-middle-class family. Content in our little world of Juhu beach evenings and *dār-dhōkdī* Sundays.

And then my little genius said a prayer, "Brother or puppy, please!" And someone up there said तथास्तु (tathāstū)[6].

At first, I refused to take on another year of breastfeeding, two years of diaper-changing, 6 years of phonics, 10 years of dance, and 18 years of round-the-clock attention. But more importantly, after loving our first so boundlessly, I wondered if we could ever love another child just as much.

I wish we'd got her that puppy.

Instead, we decided to stick to what we thought we knew how to raise i.e. a human baby. Who knew that

---

[6] Hindi for 'so be it'.

the new human baby would be nothing like our practice human baby! For the next 17 years, the Acharyas learnt to throw out our old tools and build new ones from scratch.

◆◆◆

December 21st, 2002. Krishnav Acharya was the most animated bundle of joy I had ever laid eyes on. There's a saying in Gujarati – (putr nā pag pārnā māthī), you can tell a person by their antics in the cradle. Krishnav's cradle has seen more than its fair share of his excitable movements, loud mouth, and chronic laughter. All who gazed upon him commented, "There's mischief in those eyes!" So we knew this sprightly child just wanted to run around even before he took his first steps.

Although he never really stepped if he could help it; rather, he leapt and hopped and jumped and climbed and fell and worried the living daylights out of his parents with his unstoppable activity. The house rang daily with shouts of 'Kitu, watch out!!' followed by peals of playful laughter from one least concerned about his own accident-proneness[7]. How could we have restrained him? He was a whirlwind in our lives in every sense.

While he was scaling walls, his parents were scaling up their blood-pressure. "We need an army to control

---
[7] Don't repeat my mistakes. Constant stumbling, bumping into furniture, and being accident-prone are red-flags for the risk of ADHD and/or Dyslexia. Keep an eye out for signs in your child.

him," I once said to Himanshu. My husband has been a pilot all his adult life, and perhaps never before was he more grateful to be out of the house fifteen days a month. For the other fifteen days, I single-handedly tried to make sense of these brush strokes of energy painting every corner of my house. I remember Himanshu returning home after a forty-day posting and exclaiming, "Why have you lost so much weight?" Have you seen your son?? Because I was doing the work of ten, that's why!

Why didn't I have the time to eat, you ask? Where do I even begin...

I have too many stories of my son courting disaster to fit in these pages, so here I'll restrict myself to the most memorable:

At only a few months of age, Kitu[8] was sleeping sound in his father's firm grip. When suddenly, this mischief-maker wriggled loose and jerked himself out of Himanshu's arms and landed head-first onto the floor. I had been away for work and was called home immediately. I spent the entire journey with my heart in my mouth and a prayer on my mind. I reached home

---

[8] You might read me call him all sorts of things– Kutling, Kitnav, Kaana... My apologies if this is confusing. These names are vital to the mad, glad, ridiculous spirit of our household. So whenever a name makes you think, "Wait, who is this character?", it's probably one of my children...or my husband...or the househelp. Actually, I think you'd better just take a guess.

and we rushed our sobbing child to the pediatrician, explaining with flushed faces to the doctor Krishnav's injurious thrust into the air.

Panic. Numbness. Panic. I wouldn't be surprised if waiting at the doctor's office for test results were historically certified as the most-stress inducing moment of parents' lives. Thankfully Krishnav had no internal bleeding and required medication only as a precaution. This little touch-and-go adventure shook me, reminding me (though I knew it every day) that I was raising no ordinary energy but the crazy-ball equivalent of children. I could never know what he'd do next.

At another instance, Kitu's insatiable need to splash around in every body of water sent him to the Emergency Room. On a morning like any other, I'd left a bucket to fill up under the bathroom tap. The gurgle of the flow resonated all around the house. Music to his ears, Kitu realised where the source of the sound lay – behind a half-open bathroom door.

Immediately, this two year-old decided to run to it, with no consideration for the wet, soapy floor. Afraid that her brother would slip and fall, Ashni ran to protect him, slamming the bathroom door shut before he could enter.

Well...before *all* of him could enter. Alas, Kitu had managed to stick two of his fingers into the door's hinge before it clicked shut. I came rushing to screams and tears and half my baby's middle finger hanging off his hand. We washed the blood the best we could, heaped *haldi* onto his wound, and rushed him (once again) to the hospital.

We managed to save the finger. With injection marks on his bottom and a bandaged hand, the little one came home. But only to rush right to the door where it all started! Ashni skipped three heart-beats and a breath, only to find Kitu laughing uncontrollably as he played out the accident, mocking his sister.

Everyday was a battle dance of Krishnav's antics. Team Avoid Mayhem developed a radar for trouble and kept constant watch on the trouble-maker. Team Mischief was armed with enough energy to power the city, four relentless limbs, a *kālā ṭīkā* behind his ear, and a nappy.

The teams lay in wait for the battle bugle to sound... and there it is! The pip pip pip of squeaky booties! Three against one, and the mighty warriors clash! Quick reflexes here, a little cheating there, and Team Mischief reigns supreme!

Our three vanquished heroes fought bravely but mischief has been managed. A mammoth feat that will baffle historians for eons...

For his first few years, my perpetual state was exhaustion. As much as I loved his happy-go-lucky attitude and his heart-melting laughter, running around to make sure he was safe all the time took a physical toll on me.

"Why is he so naughty, Mamma?" "When he's as old as you are now, he'll become calm and mature, I'm sure." When bogged down, I kept reminding myself to be patient. *Boys usually take longer to mature*, I lied to myself. *He's going to be fine. You're going to be fine.*

Different animals reach maturity at different ages. Horses mature around 7y-o-a, penguins at about 3. Scientists have been observing the Krishnav in its natural habitat for 17 years now, waiting for it to finally shed all its baby-feathers.

For all his early years, the Kitu has been known to squiggle out of its house when the postman arrives, running off to the neighbours. It is only to be found after much searching by a frantic mother, where it will greet her with a joyous, "Hi, Mamma! I will eat dinner with this aunty and come home, now you can go only..."

On one particularly testing afternoon, he really took the cake. Stirring a pot of daal on the stove, I realised all of a sudden that the house had been quiet for a couple of minutes. That's a couple of minutes too many for the Acharya family. I turned the stove on low and searched every room of the house, but my little racqueteer could not be found. I alerted my husband, turned off the stove, and sent out BOLO alerts to the neighbours.

"Is Krishnav at your house?"

"Did you see Krishnav leave the building?"

"Find my three year-old! Curly hair, white *ganji*, Mickey Mouse diaper! Please look out!"

When had he left? Why wasn't anyone watching him? How had I been so careless?

I could hear my heart in my throat, now dry with dread and ache. A community search continued for 40 minutes. Four different residential societies were now emotionally invested in the matter. Every house was searched, every eatery was visited, every God questioned but still nothing.

The problem was that we had been searching every space likely. Silly us! We should've been searching all places most *un*likely! We finally found him at a near-by computer coaching class, seated comfortably on the lap of an amused student, smashing keys with gay abandon. About 12 lungs breathed sighs of relief, 9 cellphones began spreading the good news, and 6 hands shot up in grateful prayer. This ad hoc rescue squad had had quite the adventure, and this full time mother had had enough.

Of course I yelled at him. What was the need to run away?? Why hadn't he at least told his sister?? And did he not think twice before walking into a strange place to mingle with strange people?? He got a sound lecture on the dangers of such carelessness.

He widened his sad eyes, nodded to show he was paying attention, and said "yes, mamma...ok, mamma" on cue. I melted as I watched the brown locks bounce on his forehead with every nod. I couldn't be angry with this cherub for too long.

All the same, because I knew he wasn't registering my reprimands anyway. I sighed[9]. While slumped over a much-needed *chai* with my head in my hands, I wondered how long I would get to rest before he gave me another anecdote to tell.

I reached out and sought advice from other parents. "You've seen him, you know how he is! How do I manage?" I asked.

Some had worthy suggestions, "Have you considered introducing him to meditation?"

Others probably picked their response from dystopian novels, "Have you tried putting him on a leash?"

He didn't have the patience for meditation and I didn't have the audacity for a leash. So for the first chapter of our lives as four, the Acharyas took to parenting Krishnav the only way we knew how – one day at a time.

---

[9] I will be sighing a lot throughout this book. For the first few years of parenting, sighs almost become punctuation marks. Mothers, can I hear 'Amen'?

CHAPTER TWO

Pappa, I Was Very in Tension...

Parenting 101, Rule #1: Don't Compare Your Children

Fact: All parents do. I have yet to meet a parent who has at no point ever wished their children would just balance the best traits of both among themselves.

At the time in my household, the metric for comparison happened to be achievements. "Achievements" in the most typically competitive sense. All those achievements that our society makes seem vital to a child's sense of self-worth – English, science, art, sports, speech and drama, UCMAS, Olympiads, tournaments, ASSET exams...the list never ends, so neither do our children's timetables.

My older one excelled in all stereotypically desirable fields. Academics, poetry, dance, and anything else thrown at her. She had superior intellect for her age, a massive appetite for knowledge, and an insatiable curiosity – she kept me on my toes! She's 21 now, and little has changed.

Krishnav, of course, had little interest in proving anything. All his adorable playfulness left him with no time to be concerned for society's ideas of "achievement". As long as he'd smiled enough by the end of the day, he was content. As long as he had eaten three giant meals and mingled with friends, he was content. And while my little rebel was out rejecting social standards of achievement, my husband and I were achieving great heights in the stress department.

In 2006, there occurred a prime example of when the polarity between my children was most evident. My older drama queen had landed an audition in an Aamir Khan Productions' film. So one day, I found myself sitting in the office reception area, waiting, wondering how Ashni was faring in the audition room.

It should be obvious by now that I was a helicopter mother, never relying on *aaya*s (nannies) and forever trying to manage every aspect of my children's lives single-handedly. Even with Himanshu on flight, I insisted on accompanying Ashnu to every round of auditions...and my refusal to hire a babysitter meant taking Krishnav along with me for hours each time. Fun.

Kitu has never had inhibitions around new spaces and strangers. Even at a formal office, he made himself instantly comfortable.

"Mamma, see I am jumping!" The springs on a couch squeak.

"What is inside??" A pantry door opens.

"Where is Ashni?" The receptionist's skirt feels a tug. "I want to see her."

He zoomed here and he zipped there, while an exhausted smile stayed tight on my face. We had barely been there a moment and I was already counting the seconds before I could take him home and put him to bed.

I couldn't help but think *I never felt like this with Ashnu*. All her life, she'd been such an accomplished child that it was getting expensive to just laminate all her certificates[10]. Here she was doing her parents proud in yet another field and not 10 metres away, this little monkey couldn't sit still long enough to construct a grammatically-sound sentence. I remember once questioning Ashni why her Sr. Kg. report card had a single A hiding shamefully among the A+s. And here, I would've been grateful if Krishnav could figure out how to button his shirt right[11].

Thankfully, the receptionist was a darling and had taken a liking to Krishnav. She directed us to a cubical usually sectioned off for the inner circle, so that Kitu would have more space to move around. We sat amongst Abbas Tyrewala and Amole Gupte, barely settling down

---

[10] Of course, we were the kind of parents who preserved every. single. one. So what if she's now a 21 y/o working professional? Who knows when we'll need to prove she won a gold at Poisar Gymkhana's butterfly drawing competition 13 years ago?

[11] Don't repeat my mistakes. This is a big red-flag for ADHD and/or Dyslexia. Keep an eye out for developmental delay signs in your child. Find out more from your pediatrician.

I'm Thoughting

when in walked Mr Aamir Khan. Without a beat lost, Kitu spilled his mind, "See, mamma! Mr. *Fanaa*[12]!"

Blood rushed to my ears. "Krishnav, shush!" I whispered, letting out a soft nervous laugh for the benefit of the adults in the room. "Why but mamma look! I'm telling you, I know him! That's *Fanaa* uncle!" The (spiritedly handsome) actor gave a good natured smile, ruffled Kitling's hair, and disappeared into another room.

The remaining present company ooh-ed and aah-ed at Krishnav's innocence. When the focus returned to Ashni's audition, Kitu snuck back into his comfort zone of hyperactivity. He'd already made one faux pas; I sat uncomfortably on edge, lest he said something drastic next time. Listening to praise for Ashni's theatrical skills, my mind didn't know how to feel. I was stretched thin between pride in one child and embarrassment in the other.

Perhaps, dear Reader, you are wondering why I was fretting so much about Kitu's antics. Perhaps you, like many others, find his monkeying around more adorable than foolish.

In retrospect, you're probably right. Krishnav behaved perhaps only twice as naughty as the average

---

[12] Khan's 2006 thriller co-starring Kajol. Remember "*Chaand sifaarish jo karta hamari...*"? Krishnav certainly did.

boy. My fault lied in that I used my daughter as a yardstick. Rather than recognise the merit in Krishnav's uniqueness, I simply chided it.

Comparing apples with oranges did nothing but make me uneasy. Regardless of the adoration people showered upon him for it, I always was fearful of Krishnav's tendency never to stick within the lines of acceptable behaviour. I felt burdened by a phantom shame that no one but I could see. For no fault of his own, my child became the object of everyone's affection and the subject of all my annoyance.

I have the privilege of retrospect today; but at this point in our story, dear Reader, acceptance will have to wait.

In case you're wondering, eventually Ashni's part in the film was scrapped. But as the universe's odd sense of humour would have it, *Taare Zameen Par* – mainstream India's introduction to Dyslexia – released sans Ashni on 21st December 2007 i.e. Krishnav's birthday!

Chapter Three

Mumma Doesn't Know Anything Only!

I'm not sure if I've already mentioned this but it's important enough to risk repeating – I was tired. I grew more tired every minute of every day as Krishnav grew louder and larger and faster. And this decided the kind of educator I was to be for my child.

Newton's Lesser-Known 4th Law: The high spirits of a mother are directly proportional to the studiousness of her child. Few things were more demotivating to me as a 21st century, formally-educated mother than watching my child shrug his academics.

There were times when I saw Ashnu sitting on the laptop, pretending to concentrate over a particularly difficult sum. and then I'd look at the mirror behind her to find that in fact she was watching one of those YouTube listicles – 'Top 10 Movie Mistakes' or *America's Got Talent* or some other media that was distinctly not homework. I despised that she was lying, of course, but I let it slide because she was a responsible girl. She got her grades and I cannot remember her ever throwing a single tantrum. I had no reason to vilify her free time.

But Krishnav, as you can imagine, did not have the same brownie points stacked up. He was often stubborn and his report card always looked like the teacher was swearing at me. As a result, it wasn't uncommon to find me voicing my annoyance. There was no justification for wasting precious time on media that wouldn't add to his knowledge.

Unfortunately, I couldn't successfully provide him with an alternative to fill the time.

Flashback to even before he began his schooling, I had grown demotivated upon knowing that he himself wasn't hungry to learn. He displayed no enthusiasm for knowledge and was seldom interested in the educative videos and books passed down from his sister. Thus, courtesy this demotivation, I lowered my standards for how much I would push him to learn. I reduced the amount of time I was willing to coax him into listening to me read. I gave in easily when he would've rather played with his cars than watch a children's film on astronomy. In essence, I gave up a little.

Each time he – this two year-old persistent in his blissful ignorance – defeated me, a thousand thoughts ran through my head. I wondered whether I was being practical and sparing myself the energy or if I was being unfair to Kitu and his development?

Wasn't the atmosphere of the house tensed each time I tried to push him? But then again, if I had put in hours of reading with Ashni, did I have the right to deny my son the same? Was I being pragmatic or was my son paying for being different? I couldn't find a black-and-white answer.

And then some relief – day schooling. When he turned 2.5[13], I could send Krishnav away for three hours a day to Jamnabai Narsee to be another maternal figure's problem. Oh, how I cherished those times of (relative) inactivity!

On the first day, this clingy one refused to let go of me for even the few designated hours in the new and unfamiliar classroom. He howled as I left, but when I came to pick him up at the end of the day, he surprised me with a beaming face.

New friends, young and old! A whole room just for play! He couldn't have been happier...but not because he was excelling, oh no! His year in Nursery was defined not by some radical shift towards being an ideal student; rather, he filled his time with pranks and tricks – all play and no work!

I was oblivious to it all. His teacher never sent home any notes or letters indicating that he was lagging behind in class. He never said much about his work at school, and I like a fool believed that the loose sheets of paper with incomplete colour-in-the-lines that he brought home were all he was expected to do.

---

[13] Since he's December-born, he was always the youngest in class. He started pre-primary at age 2.5 in a classroom of 3-3.5 year-olds, and primary school at 5.5 in a class of 6-6.5 year-olds.

At the end of the academic year, I visited the school during Open House to discuss his progress with his teacher. She said to me, "Mrs. Acharya! Your son is so loving, such a joy! He is the life of the classroom, but... he sure is a little mischievous."

"Really?" I asked, not surprised but concerned.

"Yes, but just a little. Like when I play a tape for the children to dance to rhymes, he pulls out the cassette and runs around the foyer with it, hahaha! He's adorable but we do need one teacher and two *didi*s to chase after him..."

In my head, I translated her teacher-talk to parent-speak:

"Mrs. Acharya, your son does nothing all day but run around, chatter, and distract the other children from their studies! All he wants to do is have a good time and no work!"

I smiled and made a note in my head that said 'HYPERNESS', and set it as my target for the next year. Interrupting my thoughts, his teacher continued, "...oh and also, he can't recognise the alphabet. All his peers have rushed ahead and completed reading all 26 letters. He's the only one at the bottom of the class."

I was stunned. I paused for a moment to collect my thoughts. I hope my face hadn't revealed it but my mind was only screaming one thing: Are you seriously telling me this now? At the end of the whole year?? After all your other students have *finished* learning the alphabet?

I took a deep breath and calmed my fury. There was no purpose in getting frustrated at her negligence; at this point, she had already done the damage.

And I would now have to undo it.

"Thank you for informing me, Teacher," I said with a smile, "After 8 months of being responsible for my son."

She hemmed and hawed. My mind was already sorting through the alternative teaching techniques I could think of. Somehow or another, I would get my child to read.

I went home determined to rectify this wrong. But determination didn't stem the dejection. Up until that point I had lived in a bubble, believing that it was enough to be a conscientious and vigilant mother. The news of Kitu's inability to recognise the alphabet burst this bubble, reminding me that just vigilant was no longer vigilant enough.[14]

Sometimes we forget that mothers have human limitations. And sometimes, no matter how much we push ourselves, we might not be enough for a certain situation. For no fault of our own, we come up short.

No one had told me this at the time. No one had taught me I was allowed to be patient with myself as a mother. Thus, I took Krishnav's inabilities as my failure as a parent. I decided that my primary focus for this

---

[14] Don't repeat my mistakes. Delayed reading and hyperactivity are red-flags. Check your child's developmental milestones periodically.

phase of my life was going to be making sure Krishnav caught up to and then stayed at par with his peers.

Jamnabai's time-tested print media methods hadn't grabbed Kitu's attention. It was as if he'd mastered a reflex – slamming books shut the second they were opened in front of him. By heavens, should even a whiff of knowledge seep into his brain!

So I tried every other medium I could find. I bought picture books with vibrant colours, that he categorically refused to accept as a substitute for play-time. Dr. Seuss! Barney! Amar Chitra Katha! I dramatised the stories in the books, but that too only held his attention for a few minutes. I sat him before the TV and played videos of the alphabet. Colourful anthropomorphic letters jumped on screen and danced to playful music. But the little brat! He knew this wasn't just another cartoon. Like prey smelling danger from a mile away, Krishnav sensed when something was trying to teach him and darted in the opposite direction!

Literally! He would sprint away, and I would be left to chase, grab hold of him, and sit him back down in front to face the TV, this time on my lap so he had no escape. But the gall! He'd cup his hands over his ears to block out the rhymes! The characters on the screen continued to jump around gleefully as I forced his hands away from his ears and held them tight. Now what could he possibly do?

I sat with him there, his back to me, holding his hands in place for 20 minutes. Surprisingly, he eventually settled down. He sat still without complaining when I sang along to the video, my hands never letting go of his. Then Ashni exclaimed "Mumma!" pointing at Kitu. "See, he has shut his eyes! He hasn't been watching, ahahaha!"

Where do I send in my resignation, I thought.

Two arrows, one quiver. Neither of us would budge. I kept trying different ways of engaging him and he kept finding new ways to reject them. I insisted, he resisted.

Slowly (god, so slowly) but surely, he begrudgingly learned to read the alphabet. A snippet from a song here, a flashback from a book there, the memory of a video somewhere – from a hundred different sources, he managed to recognise and store all 26 letters in his stubborn little head. Phew.

I could not have been more proud – mostly of him but also a little of myself. Yes, being a parent was my duty and I had done nothing beyond my duty. But what people won't tell you about parental duties is that they are bloody taxing. Being a single-parent for half the month to a Dyslexic-ADHD child is no joke. So every once in a while, it's important to remind yourself to appreciate that you're an effective parent because effectiveness is hard to come by. There's no guilt in taking pride in your dedication.

I visited the school again to meet his teacher, almost parading my little reader like a Mardi Gras float. *Now we'll show her*, I thought, *what my son can do with the right kind of attention!* While he of course couldn't be bothered about proving anything, I was charged.

"Kitu, point to the small 'd'..."

"Kitu, where is the big 'J'?"

"Can you trace the 'u'?"

Success at last! This little-big feat brought me hope.

◆◆◆

Hope is an intoxicating thing, isn't it? In my excitement, I enrolled him for an after-school phonetics class. But the high from Krishu's last achievement soon died down. As an established pattern now, he began to lag behind his peers in *all* academic exercises.

Fast-forward to a year later, and like a hot pan sizzling when sprinkled with water, my excitement fizzled out as Krishnav drowned me with misspelling and confused letter-casing, incomprehension and uneven spacing[15].

Now at this point, my Krishnav was showing all the typical tell-tale signs of Dyslexia. And yet, I recognised none of these. The conversation around learning disabilities is so sparse in our society that I had come to paint them all with one brush. Surely all these children were just slow, a little disinterested, a little "off". I couldn't name three distinct disabilities, I couldn't tell you what they implied, I could tell you nothing. I was clueless.

But moreover, I was prejudiced. I didn't recognise Krishnav's Dyslexia not only because I didn't know how but also because I didn't want to. As a mother, it worried

---

[15] Forgive my daughter, she's used to writing more rhyming verse than prose.

me to have my child being labeled as different. I was anxious over the stigma that would come with such a label and also over the new challenges.

I was ill-informed, which ensured I was terrified. And in my terror, I delayed getting him tested. There was no thinking about my son being different. He would come around. Everything would be ok.

So with the topic of learning-disabilities entirely taboo, we sought answers everywhere else:

"You named him after Krishna, what else were you expecting from a natkhat laal![16]"

"He's a boy. Boys just take longer to mature. Wait till he's 8 or so, they straighten up."

"What did you eat when you were pregnant with him?"

What had I eaten? *Garbh sanskār* is the belief that a child's personality forms in the womb. What the mother eats, thinks, sees, hears, all impacts the child's foundational development. Legend says that Nārad Muni taught the pregnant demon-queen Kāyadū to worship Bhagwān Nārāyan. A thousand years later (demon pregnancies, what can I tell you), Kāyadū gave birth to the legendarily pious Prahlād. He went on to bring about the death of demons in the name of Nārāyan.

In another myth, Subhadrā had listened with Abhīmanyū in her womb as Arjun explained a crucial manoeuver of war. Alas, Subadhrā fell asleep midway,

---

[16] This was Ashni's doing. The name literally translates to 'new Krishna'.

and Abhīmanyū could no longer be privy to his father's words. Decades later, this very same war maneuver proved critical to Abhīmanyū's survival. His incomplete knowledge cost him his life.

What had I eaten? What had I thought? How had I felt?

With Ashni, I had allowed the role of the mother to consume me. I was 28 and pregnant for the very first time. With all the curiosity and anxiousness of an amateur, I made sure to absorb myself entirely in succeeding at this new job. I read and read and read. I meditated and did yoga. I ate *satvik* home-cooked meals and then read some more. All my energies were devoted to completing the typical checklist for an ideal gestation.

When Krishnav came around, I wasn't an amateur and I thought I knew what to expect. With the confidence of a seasoned player, I didn't try as hard this time. I didn't think I needed to. I spent Krishnav's gestation taking care of him as any other expectant mother, but no more. Fewer books, less meditation, more laying back. Perhaps that's why second-borns are more creative go-getters – when the blanket of attention is wrapped more loosely, the little ones will make the most of the wriggle-room.

Of course, it's not the whole story but I do think my attitudes during pregnancy contributed to my children's polar-opposite attitudes towards academics. And I wasn't the only one to question if they were from two different galaxies. At the beginning of each year at school, Krishnav would find himself being taught by yet another set of teachers who had taught Ashni 4 years prior.

Invariably, they'd exclaim, "You're Ashni Acharya's brother? My my, who'd have guessed!"

And from teacher-talk to parent-speak: How does the oyster that made a pearl not know what to do now with this grain of sand?

What a folly! My grain of sand was indeed turning into a pearl. Unfortunately, I didn't recognise this; I was searching for his shine in all the wrong places...

Chapter Four

Do You Memember?

Diagnoses are scary, and my family has a surplus of them. Stage one cancer, tumours, myocardial bridges – our chemist really loves us at this point. So would the Universe have let Krishnav be? Heavens, no! Sooner or later our youngest would find something, and have his own days-of-the-week medicine box alongside ours. You know what they say: The family that medicates together, stays together!

Jokes aside, I should've been prepared for Kitling's diagnoses. By the time he was 6, we had enough indicators.

Krishnav was entirely careless with personal hygiene and possessions. He has lost and broken more water-bottles than some people have seen in their whole lives. No matter if we laminated his books with brown paper or plastic, by the end of the first month of school, they were tattered so spectacularly that I could've sold them as modern art.

He refused to talk until the ripe age of 2.5 years. and once he did, he didn't stop. He didn't adhere to a smidge of grammar or structure. He wouldn't stick to the flow of one topic when forming a sentence, instead jumping straight from Point A to Point E. He completely disregarded pronunciation, spelling, and punctuation.

He lacked any sort of interest at school, and failed standardised tests. He was unable to keep still or focus. He would leave old tasks incomplete before skipping to new ones.

> Hi didi I waunted to tell you happy rax rakshaw Bondhan and also may god help you in need which I know he will I will miss you a lot but if I have my vacations I come to meet you & and that is what I peromise you we all will miss you & may you and I remember our memories. and I still love you the way you are as for today you have got from me this letter and this little food I made for you. I will miss all that fun we had togetheir as a family when we were small all the naughtyness ess and fun stuff wee did togetheir. As I remember one insiden

Krishnav's writing, aged 13 years. Can you spot the tell-tales of an SLD?

Big. Red. Flags.

And then one of his teachers dropped a bombshell, "I think you should get him tested for dyslexia, Mrs. Acharya." Sirens wailed in the background of my mind. I knew nothing about such issues, I would've been more prepared had she come and told me he was missing an arm. But this!

"It's quite likely I passed something on to him," said Himanshu, "I had all these symptoms when I was a student. My daydreaming and lack of attention was more subtle, but I see a lot of myself at that age in him. Maybe a learning disability runs in the family...?"[17] With the utmost trepidation, I contacted the recommended expert to have my 1st-grader tested.

Clinical Psychologist and Remedial Educator Rukshan Vakil invited us for multiple tests over three days. Krishnav was beyond excited, for he thought he was there to play some fun games. Himanshu and I weren't privy to how his tests were done and were only given the final analysis. At the age of 6 years, we read the words that founded his journey as a student from then on:

> *'Superior Intelligence with good visual motor skills, which indicates that the right hemisphere of his brain is more dominant than his left. Such an imbalance often results in Learning Difficulties. Symptoms of mild Attention Deficit Hyperactivity Disorder (ADHD) indicated...'*

I was lost. I wasn't devastated but I was confused.

Today, I am so grateful for this teacher's timely advice. Our schools lack in a lot of ways but dealing with special-

---

[17] The medical community is still debating how likely it is that learning disabilities are genetically inherited. Just because you have a disability doesn't mean your child has it too. And vice versa. Causes vary from case to case so don't draw your own conclusions based on assumptions. Speak to a **Dyslexia Therapist**, **Clinical Psychologist**, or **Remedial / Special Educator** about the specifics of your child's situation.

needs children is definitely one sphere that requires massive improvement. Our children's stress levels are beyond acceptable. Anxiety, depression, eating disorders, and other behavioural disorders are difficult to recognise and more common than we'd think among students.

This teacher's vigilance probably saved Krishnav and me a lot of work. We caught his uniqueness early, and were able to identify and provide him with the special help required.

Sadly, such vigilance is neither taught nor made mandatory for our teachers – mentor figures with whom our children spend seven hours a day. As a result, students exhausted from their symptoms come home with red pen remarks from their teachers. "Lazy", "misbehaved", "academically irresponsible". Our children come home stamped with derogatory labels – labels that go a long way in shaping how they see themselves. *Different* children are told they are *less than*, when in fact, they are merely square cogs being rammed into round holes.

♦♦♦

Now that we had recognised Kitu as a square cog, we turned to the expert opinions at our disposal to determine what to do next. The agenda was to find a square hole within which this special mind would feel comfortable and would respond to learning.

The question of oral medication was almost immediately answered with a resounding 'No!' from us parents and doctors alike, given the risky side-effects[18]. Thankfully, we were assured that the non-medication therapies were known to be highly effective as well. So it was settled: We would engage Krishnav in only behavioural remedial therapies. He wasn't getting his days-of-the-week medicine box just yet.

Our schooling system sections learners by age rather than maturity, and we forget that the two do not always run side-by-side. Ideas of the "normal learning curve" are based on the archaic and fallacious assumption that there is one normal, acceptable pace at which to learn. This has an adverse effect on children's confidence.

Every child is given the same tools and expected to function no different from other children their age. As though education is a one-size-fits-all venture. Of course, this doesn't play out, and different children of the same age learn at different paces depending on the tools they are given. Those who lag begin to compare themselves to their peers, feeling inadequate and often guilty for their supposed failing in the classroom.

This leads to the fierce rat-race we see in our schools – to do the most, to be the youngest, to make a name for yourself the soonest. Encouraging ambition can be constructive, no doubt. But when we use age as a factor in competition and expect greatness from a younger and younger age group, this competition ceases to be encouraging and becomes pressuring. The stress on

---

[18] This verdict on the pros-and-cons soon changed. No treatment is black-and-white. But more on that later...

students eventually comes to hamper their progress rather than fuel healthy competition.

Recognising this, schools around the globe have begun to section children according to learning abilities rather than age. In a class, children of varied ages study side-by-side with a teacher specifically catering to their level of learning. The clear advantage here is that the teacher is able to choose their teaching technique based on the standard difficulty-level of the class.

This is impossible in a classroom of children from a single age-group with vastly different learning abilities. A teacher has to make sure those learning the fastest are not slowed down by those learning the slowest. At the same time, they have to be fair to those experiencing difficulties, and ensure they are up to speed with the rest of the class.

In Indian schools, where one teacher is in charge of 50 students at a time, how is this physically possible? How can we expect our schooling system to function if a teacher is required to explain a single concept in 10 different ways within 30 minutes?

We cannot. And thus, grouping children by age rather than ability has costs for the slowest learners in class. Teachers do not have enough time and resources to cater to each different learning level. As a result, children with special needs come home having learnt nothing, and are required to either be tutored by their parents or external tutors.

Jamnabai, like most schools today, had another solution – the Resource Room. This was a special class of a limited size. It catered to only a few children, each recognised by the school to need personal attention. Teachers were able to devote focused care in this smaller group, more effectively intervening in students' learning curves.

It allowed teachers to better understand a particular student's needs, and hence provide these special needs with special tutoring. It is a far more conducive learning environment than a jam-packed classroom, where it is easy to get distracted without the teacher noticing.

And what does ADHD love if not being distracted in class? Krishnav was promptly shifted to this new set-up.

Some teachers voiced their confusion, "I honestly cannot fathom why Krishnav is in the Resource Room. I have never found a dearth in his understanding and desire to learn. He's such a bright child!" Sigh. They weren't entirely wrong; Krishnav would sometimes surprise us with his grasp of certain concepts. Out of the blue, he'd recite a poem by rote or explain the water-cycle without mistakes! His learning was certainly not consistent, but by no means was it non-existent.

Alas, all these little gifts he gave us were verbal, never written. It was as if each time his hands tightened around a pencil, his mind let go of any information it had held. He would scribble the most illegible, incomprehensible answers during tests but come home and dictate the correct answer to a much higher degree of soundness[19].

---

[19] Don't repeat my mistakes. Disparities in written and oral knowledge are a huge red-flag for Dyslexia. Pay attention to how your child learns best.

This would not do. Hence, the Resource Room, where we would identify a different learning method that worked for Krishnav.

And we did identify a better learning method! Visual-spatial memory. In simpler terms, Kitu would remember something better if he had a visual to go with it.

He would brilliantly manipulate his Legos to create faultless masterpieces. He'd follow a robotic kit's instruction-booklet far better than he would follow a teacher reading to the class about Harappa. He'll give you dialogues verbatim from both seasons of *Sarabhai vs Sarabhai*, expressions and all. It didn't take a genius to deduce that so long as there was a visual attached, Krishnav could understand and recall anything.

Unfortunately, Jamnabai's Resource Room didn't employ Remedial / Special Educators. The RR teachers were senior teachers, with sometimes decades of experience. But they were not specially trained to assist children with specific learning disabilities.

Thus, our discovery of Krishnav's specialised need for visual-spatial material was of little use. The school did not research, acquire, and apply visual-spatial material specially for Kitu or students like him. Their methods primarily involved working a lot harder at explaining concepts to the students. They laid out simple information more often than they would for the 50-strong classrooms, especially through fun stories to grab students' attention.

This individual attention, the teachers' patience, and their kind encouragement certainly allowed Krishnav to learn faster than he would have in a regular classroom. But it is unfortunate that we couldn't provide him with the kind of specialised learning methods we knew he needed.

The silver lining? Even with non-optimal learning methods, Krishnav ended up proving one of the fastest learners in the RR. Being taken out of the hyper-competitive space of the classroom took away some of the pressure. In this more relaxed environment, he slowly ceased to resent academics!

What's more, since Krishnav's diagnosis was only borderline, he became the big fish in the little pond. Watching himself fare above his peers for the first time ever gave him a significant confidence boost[20].

Confidence is such an amazing fuel for ambition. Feeling like he *could* meant Krishnav made sure he *would*. I still remember that glowing smile on his face every time he reached a new milestone. Hearing "Well done, Kitnu!" made his face light up. That light warmed my heart as it let me know that my son finally felt capable.

"I can," he said, and I knew we were going to be ok.

---

[20] I do discourage basing one's self-confidence on a comparison with others. But at this age, such maturity could not be expected from Kitu. And if I'm being honest, I'm glad for it.

CHAPTER FIVE

But Morely, I Want to Do That...

Resource Rooms are not an uncommon feature in Indian schools. Yet, they come with a large helping of stigma. Being called a ' Resource child' was never a compliment. Naive children would ridicule Krishnav, "You are dumb or what?? Hahaha why are you in Resource?? Stupid!" Mothers too were quite misinformed, looking at me with equal parts pity and condescension in their eyes.

But I can't blame them, now can I? I too was ignorant about the nuanced minds of "Resource Children" before my child was among them. When Ashni was younger, I too remember asking her in a hushed tone, "Is he a Resource Child?" as though it was a crime, such a shameful crime.

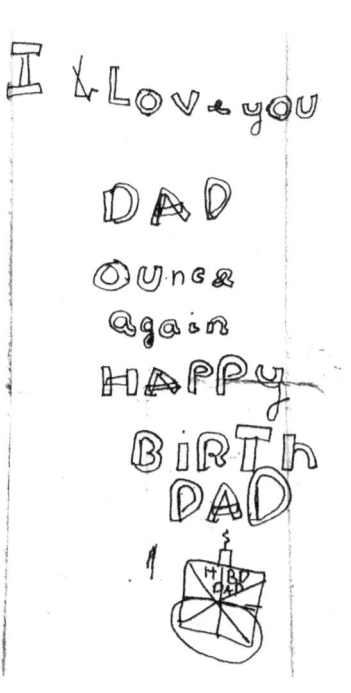

Krishnav had faced this sort of labelling and constant comparisons with his sister all his life. This hadn't laid a very strong foundation for his self-esteem. The jump in self-confidence after he joined the RR came as a relief at first. But soon, his bullies got to him once more. It didn't matter if he was performing better; Krishnav constantly doubted his academic abilities.

The only saving grace from bullying at the time was his compassion. The gullible boy barely differentiated a friend from foe. "It's ok, mumma, they can say anything. They're still my friends." He swallowed all the ridicule with a smile on his face and no malice in his heart.

I am grateful that his ability to do so did not go unappreciated. Thankfully, he had the confidence that elders loved him and recognised the incredible warmth within him. 'Pure Soul'. We heard parents and teachers alike pin him with this title, which in retrospect we value more than anything his report card could say. No amount of A+s can compete with the praise for our little one's virtues.

♦♦♦

Kitu has never had a concept of an outer circle – everyone is in the inner circle. Everyone is a friend and no one is just an acquaintance. He'd invite a ridiculous number of little boys to his birthday parties, regardless of whether or not he knew their names! "If only some people are partying, everyone else will feel bad, mamma!" Sigh.

This over-friendliness wasn't always a breeze for his mother. As any parent will know, holidays with toddlers require post-holiday holidays. On a faux-holiday before Krishnav's diagnosis, I spent the seven-hour flight sleeplessly worrying about his whereabouts.

How could I not know his whereabouts on a plane, you ask? (As I understood in retrospect,) children with ADHD find it extremely hard to be in closed spaces. Sitting still in classrooms is probably easier than sitting still in a narrow aircraft.

On this flight, Kitu accepted defeat against the seatbelt only till just after take-off. All that pent up energy then promptly pushed him off the seat to run along the aisle and greet fellow-passengers, both welcoming and asleep. With a mischievous twinkle in his eye, he made his way to the cockpit and tapped on the door. Receiving no answer, the trouble-maker took off to the other end of the aircraft, only to turn the crew's face red as he opened up pantry doors and pulled at liquor bottles.

Sigh.

By the time we'd brought him back to his seat and strapped him in, the in-flight entertainment systems couldn't compete with the spectacle he had made. Now that he had nowhere to go, he decided the passenger next to him was going to be his new best-friend.

"Hi! What is your name?...My name is Kisshnav[21]! My Mamma's name is Pinky and my Manshu Pappa is in the cockpit because he's a pilot and he's flying right now because he's wearing his uniform and my Ashni's name is Ashni, look she's sitting there because we didn't get together seats...

What are you watching?...I like cars!

Where are you going?...Are you coming with us to Thailand?...Where is your Mamma-Pappa?

What are you eating?...I don't like spicy..."

A volley of questions and information! By the end of it, the poor passenger had a lot more anecdotes and a lot less sleep than he'd signed up for. We've been lucky, though. Krishnav always finds well-tempered, understanding people to annoy. Phew! It would've been devastating for someone to have been caustic with him or complained to me.

To Krishnav, this is how human beings are supposed to interact. He doesn't do this out of a malicious desire to invade people's personal space but simply an insatiable urge to make friends with anyone and everyone. For an adult to have told him off would've been a severe blow to his confidence and brought about genuine confusion in his mind about why his niceness was being met with hostility.

---

[21] His diction wasn't perfect at this time. 'Kr' was difficult to say and so was 'h'.

And that's another thing we fail to understand when we get annoyed with special children:

Nothing they do is out of malice. They are behaving as they know best. Look close, and you will find the pure reason behind their divergences.

How was *I* on the plane, you ask? Blank. Empty. Drained of any and all damns I could give after the first few minutes. This was him all the time. I did the bare minimum to make sure he wasn't a nuisance to those around. But beyond that, I knew I couldn't single-handedly discipline him in one night. I was bereft of all energy and emotion. In retrospect, it is unfortunate how oblivious I was to the blessing of raising someone so full of love and joy.

◆◆◆

After his diagnosis, I made conscious attempts to be more accepting of his sprightly, affectionate nature. But every once in a while, I found myself trying to sandpaper my square cog, wearing him down, trying to fit him into the round hole. Himanshu and I would wonder aloud to one another, "Why can't he just sit still? Why can't he just be silent?" But what we were really saying was 'Why can't he just be like other kids? Why can't he walk the line?'

Through grades three and 4, we saw a marked improvement in his academics with the help of the Resource Room staff. He began to display a genuine urge to follow instructions and perform better in a school set-up. He gradually grew less and less disinterested in reading, and made a greater attempt to correctly recognise, understand, and pronounce larger words.

"That was a great effort, Kitu!" We tried to encourage him as best we could, to make sure he knew his work was worth continuing.

But like any journey, a stretch of calm waters must never be taken to harken a smooth sea. These initial improvements were great strides, but Kitu still wasn't there yet. His writing was still often illegible; his 'b's were still 'd's; his full-stops had gone to take a walk at some point and we had never heard from them again.

Worst, his passion to learn began and ended at being able to score just enough at school. Essentially, he wasn't interested in *learning* as much as he wanted to be done with *studying*. And we cannot blame him. All his life, he had been judged primarily based on his marksheet. It was what most authority figures around him fixated upon. Such an attitude cannot garner a joy for learning, only a desire to score, if for no other reason than just to shut up those telling you to score.

Like a child with a bad grade in spelling, Himanshu and I wrote the same sentence in our minds again and again, trying to etch it in memory:

Morale > Marks
MORALE > MARKS
MORALE > MARKS!!!!!

But our conditioned ideas were difficult to uproot. We were angry at ourselves, as if raising a child was a project and we had failed. In trying to make him a 'successful' child, we forgot to enjoy raising our son. Rather than celebrate all the things he was, we fussed over all the things he wasn't.

To combat his dispassion for learning, we made him dabble with sports. From tennis to karate, we attempted to hone his focus in a physical activity, hoping it would translate to cognitive activities. At this point in the story, dear Reader, I feel like you have an idea of the pattern such ventures with Krishnav take. So it doesn't take a genius to guess that we managed to score very very high, if our goal was to quit as many sports as possible within two years.

First there was football. I stood by the field to watch how he was coping. He ran along the white chalk circumference like he was asked, looking at me while panting as if to say, "How could you?? And to your own son???" I paid no heed to the drama-king.

I watched the toddlers in their adorable jersey shorts line up one after another to take turns kicking a ball towards the goal. Somewhere in the middle of the line, Krishnav awaited his turn.

Minutes passed as I watched the other children, and I suddenly realised how long it had been and still Krishnav hadn't gotten his turn. It made no sense. There were hardly 10 kids in front of him; why was he taking so long to reach the front of the line?

And then I noticed. Unbeknownst to the coach, this sly little thing kept running to the back of the line each time he moved up a few positions, never once making it to the ball! Sigh. I sank my head into my palms. So football was off the list.

Then came swimming. When he wasn't trying to skip class over a phony stomach ache, Krishnav kept the lifeguards on their toes. Not because he was likely to drown, no. To be fair, he was and still is quite a decent swimmer. Rather, the pool staff kept an eye on him to make sure he wasn't surreptitiously drifting away from the rest of the class. "*Arre* Kisna! Where are you going! Finish the lap! Swimming करने से ज़्यादा तो रुक रहे हो (*karné sé zyādā tō ruk rahé hō*)![22]"

The reason I mention what can only be described as the high blood-pressure epidemic among coaches across Mumbai, is because looking back upon these stints have made me see them in a whole different light. What's common among these incidents[23] was that Krishnav gleaned friends, laughs, and love wherever he went. He splashed around with the littler ones in the kiddy pool, showing them how to make the most of the fountains. He laughed with grandfathers between their laps and told the lifeguards about his week. He never swam like a professional, but all the while he was practicing a skill far rarer.

◆◆◆

---

[22] Hindi for, "You are stopping more than you are swimming!"

[23] ...besides tens of new and now useless specialised shoes. Big Sports and their manufactured needs, I tell you...

Capitalist society has a very set understanding of value. We have made for ourselves a system that knows only how to value people for how much they can contribute to an economy – how much they can earn, what skills can be put to "productive" use. We laud excelling at the sciences, landing a high-paying job, or being able to live in the posh part of posh cities.

I've seen parents of high-achieving students sit silent as their children bully and taunt. I've seen mothers flaunt medals but say nothing about how their children treat other human beings. Sure, the same kids will end up with money and medals in the future too. But what of seemingly 'uneconomical' virtues of humanity?

Productivity regardless of virtue.

If this was the natural and absolute yardstick for a life well-lived, then what can we say of the lives of PWDs? Is a soul unimportant because it is uneconomical? Is my child's life of less "value" because they can't compete in productivity with abled bodies?

Like Himanshu and I, society too has made the mistake of forgetting what PWDs have while focusing on what they lack. You will find no textbooks teaching you to calculate the value of virtue in society. No professor will tell you that kindness, compassion, empathy – despite and probably *because* they cannot be concentrated as capital – are crucial to the functioning of our global system. No one will remind you that your special-needs child doesn't need to be "productive" to be enough.

Write it five times in your notebooks and say it aloud, Parents:

A life of goodness is a life good enough.

Back to Krishnav, I am blessed to have a son who lives by Jane Austen's words, "I have no notion of loving people by halves, it is not my nature."

CHAPTER SIX

No Fault of Kārtikéya's

A Small Interruption from Ashni

Parents have favorites. We know you never want to but c'mon, you know you do. And kids are not oblivious to this. You may tell us and yourselves, "Mamma-Pappas love all their babies equally!" but your subtle preferences are all too cumulatively palpable. But don't worry! We get it.

I'm sure Pārvatī loved her *agraj* Kārtikéya, her firstborn with all her heart. But our mythologists make it abundantly clear the favorite in the family was the *anuj*, the second-born. She made him from the paste from her own skin, moulded him with her own hands, prayed life into him with all the divine power her mind could muster. Ganésh was, in the most intimate sense, a part of his mother's *being*.

And then the torment of having to find your son slain! The tragedy of Ganésh's decapitation must've weighed on Pārvatī's heart like a boulder. She alone knows how she held herself together through the long and aggravating process of gathering the wise men of the heavens and compelling them to restore her son's life. One can only imagine the agonising wait while the gods brought the elephant's head to fit Ganésh's body, and the pure joy of watching her son open his eyes once more! After such a whirlwind of emotions, can one blame a mother for a special attachment to this son?

As unfair as it may seem to Kārtikéya, I can sympathise with Pārvatī. Imagine if through all of Ganpati's ordeal, the older one came tugging at his mother's dupatta, wondering why she wasn't in the mood to take up his homework or play Scrabble with him. Imagine having to make your first child feel secure while being perpetually in anxiety over your second (what with him being a little headless and all).

When raising a special needs child, it's only natural to be wrapped up in all there is to take care of just so they lead a smooth functioning life. For no fault of our own, us Kārtikéyas of the world may grow up feeling a little abandoned and a little insecure. This question plagued Mom as it does many mothers of Dyslexic children all the time: How to make sure your other child doesn't feel like *the other* child?

Being the first child in the whole generation on either sides of the family, I was accustomed to undivided love for the first 4 years of my life. By the time I had reached my preteens, I had to learn to share my parents with quite a time-consuming little brother.

Earlier, Dad used to be off flying 20 days of 30. For 2/3rds of the month, Mom was a single-parent with a

Dyslexic-ADHD child, which is hard enough. On top of that, she was also expected to run the house, have a career, and parent her older one. But like everyone else, she had just 24 hours a day, 4 limbs, and one brain – there were only so many places she could reach. As a consequence, I found myself having to do a lot of maturing on my own.

First off, I had to be ok with double-standards.

I remember the night of a dinner we'd hosted for the extended family. I couldn't have been older than 11-12 years, which puts Krishnav at about 7. The guests started pouring in and my excitement with the night waned. Who wants to make polite conversation with elders who only talked about people I didn't know and in words I didn't understand? I asked my father if I could watch TV while the guests talked amongst themselves, and he immediately reprimanded me for my ill-manners. "Good children don't start the TV when guests come home. Go help your mother with serving the table," he said. I did as I was told.

An hour or so later, I was laddling rice into the elders' plates when Krishnav ran up to the table and said, "I'm bored, can I watch some TV?" Without flinching, Dad agreed. It may sound silly but to 12 year-old me, the hypocrisy displayed in that moment was astounding. I stopped laddling the rice, placed the bowl on the table, and glared down at him in rage. The three other men at the table stopped chewing to look confused at my shamelessness. "What?" Dad said, "Because of the TV? *Bachchā*, he's younger than you are."

"You're the older one." was my parents' mantra throughout my childhood. Krishnav would run around in public spaces, being loud and unruly while I was expected to be perfect – back straight, hair pulled back, soft voice, all smiles. Krishnav threw tantrums and demanded attention while I never questioned my mother's word. So when guests came home, Krishnav was allowed to make mischief with the other kids while I had to learn to be a good host.

I grabbed the rice bowl and stormed back to the kitchen. *He's going to be the younger one all his life!* I thought. *Is he never going to be expected to mature at all? What sense does that make?*

♦♦♦

Looking back now, I understand. Not only was Krishnav younger but he could not be disciplined the way I could. I could be told not to watch TV and I would oblige. Due to his hyperactivity, Krishnav needs more elaborate, longer-term instructing for most disciplining even today. It took several years before he satisfactorily learned to do even simple things like brush and bathe himself, as is standard for special-needs children.

So Dad didn't tell him not to watch TV because he would've simply thrown a tantrum. What Krishnav needed was a repeated explanation and demonstrations of what it means to be a good host, which were not possible instantaneously. But to 12 year-old Ashni, this was not as lucid then as it is now, and I was mad.

The cumulative effect of years of such discrepancies in my parents' behaviour towards Krishnav and I was that I learnt to live and grow independently. They had not a clue that I had developed an illness; I pulled myself from diagnosis to convalescence without their knowledge. I chose not to involve them because one heavily dependent child is enough to occupy all your mental capacity.

When they did find out, they were devastated. Even today, when I'm all healthy and have their unwavering support, they still feel guilty. And this, I think, is all too common among parents – guilt.

I didn't do this.

I wasn't around for that.

I didn't catch this.

I didn't change that.

Dear Parents,
Please chill.

– Thanks and regards,
Your BP.

My Mom had a household, a career, and a special-needs child to be concerned with.

My Dad had a job that kept him out of the country for 2/3rds of my life.

Parents, *you have lives outside your children.*

You cannot always be cognizant of our ups and downs. You will miss out on several things throughout our lifetimes. Knowing you cannot guard every aspect of your child's lives is part-and-parcel of being a guardian.

Yes, I did feel like a Kārtikéya. Many of us will. But the Pārvatīs of the world cannot be blamed. There's only so much a human can do.

> *Well, why didn't Acharya leave work for later?*
> *Shouldn't your children come before your career?*

She did leave work for later. Mom's career would've taken off so much faster had she not been as involved with Kitu and I as she was.

She started practicing as a Graphologist when Kitu was 3 y/o but didn't seek her first big contract till he was 9. She refused to go to an office full-time so she could help Krishnav study. She became Marshall Goldsmith's 'Global Leader of the Future' only when he turned 14, and got her ACC certification when he was 15. We've heard it all through his life, "Not yet, Kitu still needs me."

Even today, she spends not more than 6 hours a day on her career, and the rest of 18 hours making sure I've eaten and Kitu hasn't overeaten, making sure the house is clean and the *dhōbī* is paid, making sure my Naani isn't over-cleaning and my Daadi isn't over-cooking…I can really go on and on.

> *Well, maybe she should've done more. Put her*
> *career completely on hold to make sure both of*
> *you were ok.*

Women don't forfeit their right to personal growth when they become mothers.

Maybe she just wasn't good at multitasking.

Have you ever run a household, Imaginary-Side-Narrator-I-Created-to-Make-a-Point-About-Working-Mothers?

No, but...

Good. જેનું કામ જે કરે (*jénū kām jé karé*)[24]. Now don't interrupt with your baseless judgement of a situation you've never experienced and let me conclude this chapter.

Sorry.

The bottom line is being a mother is consuming and being a mother to someone with special needs is all-consuming. The purpose of this interruption is to remind the Pārvatīs that cutting down on your involvement with your Kārtikéyas doesn't make you an unfair mother.

Even without special-needs kids, no parent can do an absolute job. Your children are going to fall, feel insecure, and go through horrible things you might not be able to help with. It's an inalienable part of parenting, and most often we're stronger for it.

I have no resentment for the decisions my parents have made for us, nor for the growing I've had to do

---
[24] Gujarati for 'don't comment when you're not qualified to'.

without them. I may have wanted all the attention but Krishnav needed it. No fault of Kārtikéya's but also no fault of Pārvatī's. C'est la vie.

End of Small Interruption from Ashni.

CHAPTER SEVEN

Little a Bit Medicine

Remember when I said that our family has an affinity for pills? Our dining table looks like Patanjali, Baidyanath, and Cipla had a carboot sale. And soon enough, it fell on Krishnav's shoulders to carry on the family tradition...

Epileptic Negative Myoclonus

It's basically a brief seizure. Your muscles stop working for a second, and any activity they may have been engaged in will cease. There is no consensus on the cure.

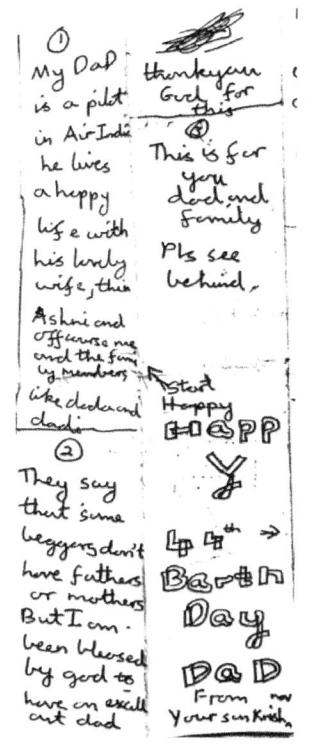

By the time he was 9 y/o, we were used to Krishu being clumsy. He tripped and bumped into things often[25], dropped gadgets and spilled food. We presumed it to be regular kiddy hyperactivity. But this was different.

Kitu was on his way to an after-school class when he tripped without warning. Not thinking much of it, he helped himself up, dusted himself off, and continued onward.

When he sat down to work, his teacher noticed that the *bachcha* wasn't able to meet the tip of the pencil with the surface of the paper. For just a moment, his hands would stop short just as he was about to complete the action, and then he'd continue. So brief, in fact, were these spasms that they could've easily gone unnoticed.

"What happened, Krishnav *beta*? Are you tired?"

"No, Ma'am. I just blanked out."

We brought him home, hoping nothing worse was yet to come. We asked him what he was feeling but we couldn't put our finger on what exactly had happened. No one said the word 'fit'.

We had just decided to let the matter rest, to see how things panned out, when Kitu sat on the table for his meal but couldn't lift his spoon. I saw a glaze of emptiness wash across his eyes, only to vanish in a split second. This was not just fatigue.

Cut to a few hours later, we found ourselves in the office of a reputed pediatric neurosurgeon. We were bracing for the worst, our faces blanched in worry. As

---
[25] Don't repeat my mistakes. Speak to a pediatric neurologist about red flags of developmental delays in your child's daily movements.

a parent you are either brave or you put up a brave face. We kept our smiles up for Krishnav, never wanting him to fear there was something wrong with him.

"Alright, my dear boy, keep your eyes open and raise your hands...very good. Now try to point them at each other...wonderful. Now shut your eyes and take a few steps forward..." After the preliminary exercise-based tests, the doctor recommended conducting VEEG and MRI scans. The Video-EEG takes several days, since it must map the brain's activity while active, asleep, and seizing.

♦♦♦

So off to the hospital for a weekend, it was. Guess who was most excited. Away from the towering walls of school, without Mamma-Pappa's nagging to complete homework, surrounded by fascinating instruments, odd bots, and shiny screens – I don't think I have seen anyone so awestruck with reclining beds and sterile gowns.

And that proved to be an issue. Giggling as the doctor fixed several electrodes on his head, Krishnav was so excited that he refused to sleep. Can you imagine this boy! "Kitu, we need to monitor your sleep, na? Just try shutting your eyes for a few minutes." The technician practically begged. We tried everything – distracting him from the excitement with a story, reading, sleeping next to him. Nothing. Finally, we medically-induced his sleep and the thankful doctors got on with their jobs.

After a day of listening to rhythmic beeps and staring at monitors I didn't understand, we were done[26]. A real sucker for the spotlight, he had thoroughly enjoyed being the center of affection from us and the hospital staff. On the way out, he told the doctor, "This was fun! I'm going to tell all my friends about it!"

The MRI process to follow sounded like a nightmare for anyone with ADHD – an enclosed space in which Kitu would be expected to lie still, without commenting every seven seconds on how cold the floors are and why do doctors wear green shower caps and what's the blue flashy thing…

And God sent us an angel in the guise of the resident doctor. Her name escapes me at the moment but it was as if she had been made for children like Kitu. They clicked instantly, sitting on either sides of her desk laughing in unison, like mirrors. They bounced incessant chatter against one another, exuding joy that lit up both their faces with a cherubic radiance. The comrades walked hand-in-hand to the MRI theatre, gay and oblivious to the set of parents praying behind them.

"When you go into the tunnel, just shut your eyes, okay? You'll be out in just a few minutes, brave boy!"

"Ok but can my Pappa hold my hand?"

"Of course! He'll be in there with you." With a comforting sisterly air, she assuaged all his and my fears.

---

[26] Ashni takes special pleasure in the fact that we had to snip off tufts of his hair when simply peeling away the electrodes got too painful. To be fair, he did look a little ridiculous.

"Tell me, kiddo, what are you going to do when we're done with your scan?"

"Eat. Nurse aunty didn't give me breakfast." We laughed.

He went into the machine with the air of a loyal disciple, didn't move a muscle throughout, and left the room beaming. I was proud, as though he'd just won an Olympic gold in 'Competitive Laying Down'. So he *was* capable of stillness! He walked out of the theatre and up to the doctor, and said, "It's lunch time. I have to have two meals now." And he did. Lord knows I would've given him two meals for every meal if it meant this level of discipline.

The next day, we went about our day entirely distracted, waiting for his results to come in and ease our trepidation. But when they did grace us, the results only replaced the anxiety of not knowing what was wrong with the anxiety of not knowing what to do about what was wrong.

"...temporary breaks in brain activity and motor coordination..."

Sure enough, Kitu had ENM. What now?

♦♦♦

Medication. We were told it might affect his education, but we only laughed. That was the least of our concerns, for it was the oldest of our concerns. Right now, all we cared about was for Krishnav to be healthy. And so we began for the first time with oral medication. And even then he wasn't allowed to leave the house unaccompanied and we observed him 24x7.

The first medicine Krishnav was put on, let's call it 'ZP', stopped the epileptic attacks. We never saw another episode. But it also started to have very obvious side-effects. The most obvious one was that Krishnav became quieter. The kind of silence that only prevailed when he was away now filled the house despite his presence. He lost his excitement, lost his former effervescence through mundane life. He became listless – regular for anyone else but surprising for someone with his spirit. Something wasn't right.

The dam broke when one day Kitu walked out of his room crying. Caught off-guard by his unprovoked tears, Himanshu and I rushed to him asking what happened. "I don't know, I just feel horrible," he replied. We sat down with him, trying to help him decipher why he was feeling the way he did, but to no avail. Then all of a sudden, he said, "It's the medicine. It's making me sad."

No idea how he had such insight but thank god he did. We checked with our doctor and they confirmed – ZP did have the potential to dull patients' moods. No way were we going to allow Krishnav's light to be dimmed by a pill. This was too high a cost to pay.

The alternative was another drug, let's call it 'PR'. We gave PR a shot and within no time, we saw Kitu return to his regular self. Not only did the epilepsy never return but also there was no more dullness, no more fits of crying, no more sad outbursts.

Moreover, we were ecstatic with PR's effect on Krishu's VEEG results. After a month of the medicine, we returned to the hospital for the required re-examination, and viola! None of the abnormalities in the initial test had persisted! A perfectly regular scan, you could never have guessed this brain had seized just over a month ago.

Our doctor was speechless. He ran the results by other doctors just to be certain this wasn't an optimistic mistake. "We have never seen such a recovery," he said. We didn't truly understand how peculiar Kitu's case was till the doctor requested our consent to present Krishnav's case at an upcoming international doctors' conference.[27]

But all was not hunky-dory. Kitu had to take PR for the next two years, which affected his academics significantly. Extended tutoring, more yelling, and dropped scores awaited us till he turned 14 y/o. When he reached the 9th grade, we reached breaking point...

---

[27] We consented, and the conference came to no conclusion about why Kitu had recovered so miraculously. Our ordeals are always short lived.

Chapter Eight

Don't Undera... underamamestimate Me!

From the 5th to the 8th grade, we struggled with Krishnav's low performance at school. In that time, we made one of the biggest parenting mistakes since Duryodhan. Bribery or, if you want to feel a little less evil, 'incentivising'.

It's a constant for most of our lives in some form or another. Your government *bābū* won't register a complaint without *bakshīsh*. God won't reverse your stock losses without barefoot walks to Siddhivinayak.

The result is a loss of a sense of duty. We begin to do things not each time we should but only when we see an incentive.

Of course there are many behaviours for which incentives are legitimate, like favours. But these behaviours are transactions, not duties. But to incentivise duties is to quash their value of good-faith.

For example, an electrician must necessarily be given their due fees after they've fixed your lights. That is a transaction, since they are not obligated to help you. But imagine a world where your doctor demands an incentive to be sober when performing your mother's surgery! Sobriety during work hours is their duty; how ludicrous it is to need an incentive!

In sum: We cannot put a price on the behaviours of good-faith that keep society's wheels smoothly in motion. If individuals begin to demand incentives for their duties, we would end up in an immoral dystopia.

◆◆◆

And the same with the lil ones. We incentivise their duties as though they do us a favour by being model children.

"Please stop harassing me while I work! Go watch some TV."

"Fine, I'll give you chocolate if you finish all your *rōṭī-sabzī,*."

"If you score better next time, we'll buy you a new phone."

And then they expect chocolate after each meal and a new gadget after every test. By the end of it, we've conditioned children to believe that the world must reward you before you do no more than your job.

Unfortunately, this insight only comes with the luxury of retrospect. From the 5th to the 8th grade, bribing became our go-to for getting Krishnav to drop his resistance to duties, namely studying. Each time he refused to look at a textbook, we'd bait him with the promise of 30 minutes of TV-time. "Just finish this last sum, *bétā*," you'd hear Himanshu say, "Then you can go watch whatever you want, I won't say a thing."

When 30 minutes stopped doing the trick, it became harder and harder to keep his attention. Break-lengths kept increasing while his scores remained largely stagnant. Each time Kitu came home with a paper, we'd sit down and have a long talk revisiting his screen-time privileges.

"These scores are not acceptable. You can't take two hours of TV per day if you're going to be scoring like this. Your TV-time is reduced to one hour. Show us better results and you can watch as much as you'd like." Needless to say this model was not sustainable.

Furthermore, when bribery didn't work, we simply gave in to each of Krishnav's tantrums. Krishnav eats his feelings, and all through his life it has been a task to control his diet. Whenever someone would bring home sweets, I would hide them among the flour containers or in the vegetable cabinet of the refrigerator. How else would they last beyond a minute in Krishnav's hands?

I'd pack fruits, nuts, and other healthy options for his school snack. They would come home untouched. He'd storm into the house, annoyed that he hadn't eaten anything since morning, demanding chips, *kachori*, or some other fried heart-clogger.

Each day he would demand unhealthy snacks and each day I would refuse at first. We would get into an argument, wondering why the other won't see sense.

I would tire of this daily battle and eventually give up. "Here," I'd say, "Eat this!. Do whatever you want, because that's what you do anyway!"

For years, we would have the same fruitless (geddit?) discussions around what he should eat and how much, always ending with me capitulating. I would give in, sigh, and then watch as my son defied me and any logic. My blood-pressure would rise as I would watch him gulp down ice-cream by the spoonful. Again, an unsustainable parenting style.

♦♦♦

By the 8th grade, we'd had enough. We switched tactics, tried to bring back his sense of duty towards his education as well as his body.

We've swapped the carrot for a better, organic, GMO-free locally-sourced carrot – something I like to call 'emotional engineering[28]'. We've begun to speak to Krishnav about his duties in a manner that taps into the parts of his conscience he values most i.e. making his parents proud. The last thing he would want to do intentionally would be disappointing Himanshu and I. We know he adores us and feels terribly guilty when he defies us. So we use that against him.

When we are yelling at each other like adversaries, this adoration and guilt doesn't surface. When

---

[28] Of course, it's a euphemism for 'blackmail'. We don't want to feel manipulative, now do we? But what really is *all* disciplining if not 'engineering'?

demanding that he performs his duties, we come across as the enemy, against whom he could only win if he was defiant. But now – when phrasing his behaviours as a way to make sure he didn't disappoint his parents – we leverage that adoration and guilt to our advantage.

A before and after looks a little something like this:

Giving-In / Bribery	**Emotional Engineering**
Fine, don't help Mamma in the kitchen, you spoilt brat!	*If you don't help Mamma out with the vessels, we'll be quite disappointed.*
Study for another half hour, only then can you go play gully cricket.	*If you study for another half hour, we'll be really proud of you.*
Alright, alright! Go take another 15 minutes of TV! Just stop chewing my brains!	*If you lie to us about your TV-time, we will believe we have failed as parents.*
Be the kind of student you're supposed to, then I'll consider wasting my money on your stupid headphones.	*If you don't buy these headphones you don't need, we'll be very happy with how maturely you've begun to make your decisions.*

The bribery approach only serves to make the child dependent on incentives. That's not how the real world outside your household will treat them. The emotional engineering approach makes the child very aware of the onus on them to be good and fulfill their duty. It's also less antagonising; your child won't be fuming at you after.

Thus, we've found that the fruit lies in patience. It's time and effort-consuming but far more sustainable in the long-run to appeal to Kitu or any other child's conscience.

Of course, this is not a linear process. Every once in a while, we still find that it saps our energies to convince him to eat right or put his phone away before bed. But most often, in moments like these when one of us is about to give up, the others in the house are thankfully prompt to swoop in. It takes a village to raise a child – *everyone* in the house needs to be involved in correcting behaviors through emotional engineering.

Slowly but surely, he is…no, the whole household is trying. How long will it take before we undo the effects of years of conditioning? We cannot say. But what we know for sure is that we're on the right track. As I always say for my family, we never fail – we either succeed or we learn.

CHAPTER NINE

When I Grow Up, My Height Will Be Big!

When Krishnav touched the 6th grade, his studies were beginning to occupy my time almost as much as they occupy this book. Everything needed revision, and every revision needed a nap.

Krishnav's Achilles heel was writing tests. When tested on a subject orally, he'd recite anything assigned to him with ease and flair. But if you asked him to write what he had just said, you'd get a sheet filled with something that most resembled hieroglyphics.[29]

When he'd come home after writing a paper, we would ask, "How was it?" and each time his reply was consistent, "*Arre* what an amazing paper! I knew everything!" But of course, when our eyes eventually met the marksheet, we would wish we'd turned blind sooner.

---

[29] Does your child do this too? Discrepancies in written and oral answers are a big red flag for learning disabilities.

I'm Thoughting

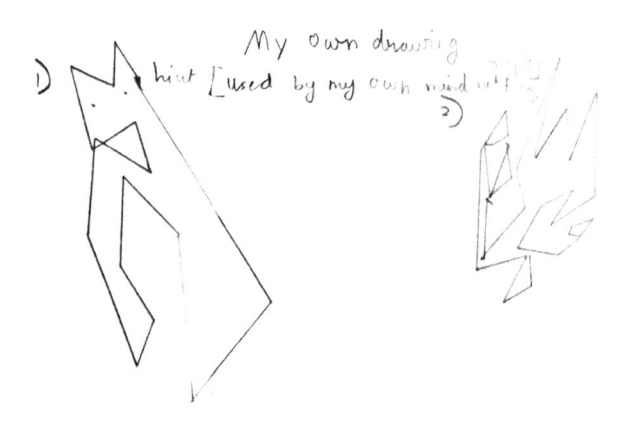

60-something percent was a good day. Gaping holes in his transcript would reveal that while the ABC and XYZ of the answer were present, D-to-W had been eaten up. "Where is the rest of it? Didn't you know it?" He'd simply say, "I don't know what happened. I thought I wrote everything!"

Sigh.

◆◆◆

We decided to give remedial education a shot. Experts consistently have backed remedial therapy as the only long-lasting strategy towards mitigating the symptoms of Dyslexia and Dysgraphia. Therapists are hard to come by since few practice certified techniques. But we were told the search is worth it. The method ostensibly has an impressive track record in managing SLDs.

Unfortunately, Krishnav was not one of those students.

We tried multiple practitioners claiming to be remedial specialists. One such is worth mentioning: A 30-something year-old dire disciplinarian, she wielded her tongue like a spear. There was no warmth in her teaching, no joy in her work, and no reason for an attention deficient student to want to spend 90 continuous minutes listening to her. Her tone was caustic and her methods were inflexible – exactly the opposite of what children respond to.

The whole affair was quite painful, and as you can imagine Krishnav didn't take to her at all. Even after months, we saw no results. Besides Krishnav not being a good fit for her, she wasn't a good fit for her job. If there's anything my husband and I have learnt in raising Krishnav is that love and patience is the key. Harsh words can never yield results, only antagonise.

As you can imagine, his report cards were a consistent mess. But what most raised my eyebrows was his self-evaluation. On one occasion, his class teacher asked each of her students to jot down what they thought of their test scores through the months i.e. self-assess their trajectory.

Krishnav submitted his:

60% = Excellent!

40-50% = Very good!

35% = Good.

<35% = It's ok, try again next time:)

Hilarious as always, but the underlying problem won't disappear in our laughs. Unfortunately, we needed him to score well, regardless of how skewed we thought the grading system was.

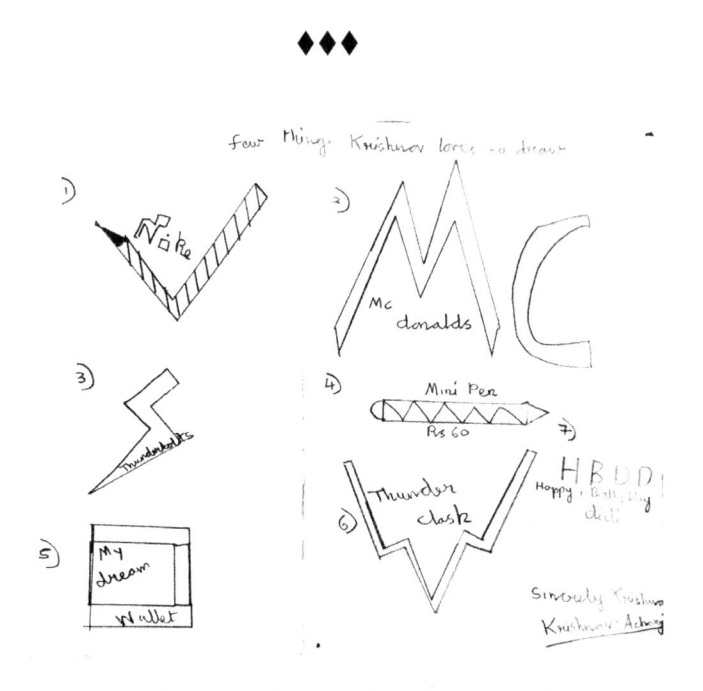

◆◆◆

[Handwritten sketch: "Four things Krishnav loves to draw" — 1) Nike logo, 2) McDonalds M/C, 3) Thunderbolts, 4) Mini Pen Rs 60, 5) My dream wallet, 6) Thunder clash, 7) HBD! Happy Birthday didi. Sincerely Krishnav, Krishnav Achrey]

We know that the kind of standardised universal education we have today is not inclusive for children who are in any way different – physically, intellectually, or creatively. In formal education, to be different is to be lesser. There is but one yardstick for success and every child is expected to fit it.

This is a complete denial of the uniqueness of each individual learner, which especially affects students of subaltern groups (lower castes, tribes, women) and the disabled community (especially if of lower caste, tribal, or female).

Quoting a paper mentioned in Dr. Abha Sur's *Dispersed Radiance: Caste, Gender, and Modern Science in India*:

> *"...the principle point is that measures of scientific performance admitted of only a single scale, according to which, to be different was to be lesser. Under such circumstances, the hope of equity, indeed the very concept of equity, appears to depend on a disavowal of difference."*

This holds true for education as a whole today. In simpler terms, the world of education has come to accept only a singular kind of success, and any deviations are immediately relegated to the realm of failure. If you want to advance, you must conform.

There's a gorgeous painting called *The School of Athens* by Raphael. You must've seen it at some point. It's the one where Plato and Aristotle walk towards the audience from the center of the canvas, a horde of pensive looking white men all around them.

Plato points upwards just as his *Theory of Forms* looks upwards. He posits in this theory that there exists in the abstract a realm of universal 'Forms'. This is where there exist the perfect and universal examples of anything and everything you'd find in the human realm – Forms of the perfect Horse, the perfect Triangle, the perfect Slave. For Plato, the goal of human society was to mimic everything to match the Forms. Earthly horses must strive to conform to the Form of the perfect Horse.

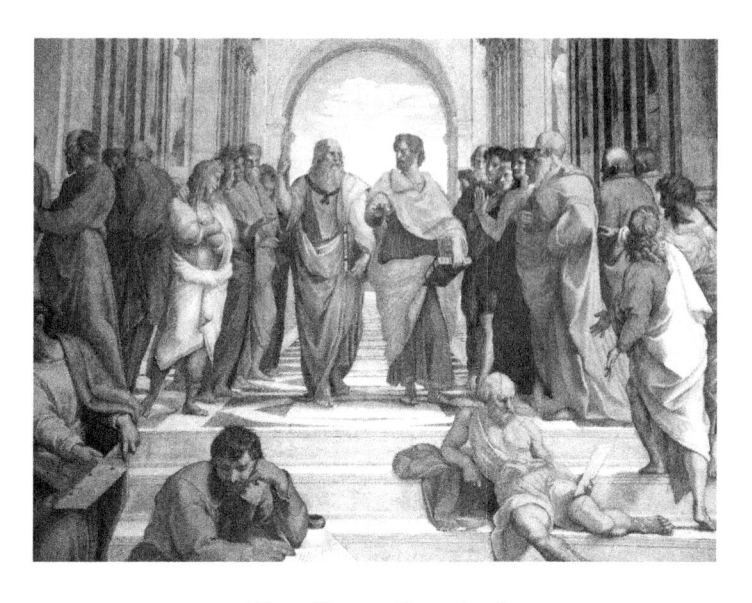

Album/Oronoz/SuperStock

Sounds familiar?

Right beside Plato, Raphael paints an Aristotle gesturing forward. Aristotle's theory focuses on this present realm rather than an abstract one. He challenges Plato, and denies that there exists any universal Forms – no perfect Horse for earthly horses to conform to. Rather, he focuses on the attributes of things that humans can actually perceive with our senses.

Instead of trying to fit all things in the human realm to some abstract Form, he believes the Form is intrinsic to everything. In simpler terms, there is no universal Form of the Horse; rather, the form of the horse lies in *every* earthly horse. So the goal of the earthly horse is no longer to fit some ideal; rather, it is to realise that something makes *every* horse a horse in their own right.

Industrial education has given in to the idea that each student is meant to fit the perfect Form of the student. There's no widespread modern-day Aristotle to challenge mainstream education, to compel us to understand how each student is a student in their own right.

Parents, there is no perfect universal Student. There is only the unique studiousness that is inherent to your unique child.

And if you ask me, without the idea of a perfect Student, there can be no concept of "learning disabilities". Some children learn differently. Once we accept that, we understand that these children are not deficient just because the world made an education system that excludes them. The deficiency lies in the system that claims to be universal but fails to accommodate some of the world's greatest minds.

♦♦♦

I didn't want to teach my son to conForm. I didn't want him to believe that the only way to be considered worthy of some sort of standing in the world is to deny himself any creativity. It saddens me to think of a system that views education as a somehow sanctimonious process – so perfect that not aligning with it indicates a major flaw in *you*.

What an unforgiving world that doesn't change education to suit the person but tries to change the person to suit the education?

And yet, we knew that if he wanted to get into a good college, he'd need some semblance of success in formal education. Against all logic and fairness, he would have to include himself in an exclusionary system.

A possible compromise? ICSE allows children with disabilities to engage a 'scribe' – a student (one year academically junior) responsible for writing answers that the examinee dictates. This way, learners with SLDs can rely on their strength i.e. oral answering to give an otherwise written test. We had the option of doing Krishnav's examiners a favour and replacing his handwriting with that of a neurotypical student. But we never could bring ourselves to do it. Being assigned a scribe also meant being assigned the stigma that comes with. While Kitu would have done much better in tests, his confidence would have dipped. We were worried about peers teasing him for needing assistance.

Our worries were not without precedence. While engaging with other mothers at school, I had often heard some make comments or display tight, uncomfortable expressions when they'd find out a particular child had a scribe. As though proof of knowledge given orally is less legitimate than proof of knowledge given in writing.

Unfortunately, I succumbed at the time. But now, to all these uncomfortable faces, I ask:

Why this culture of shame in admitting we need help? Should we start being embarrassed when taking care of other deficits like vitamin deficiencies or amputated limbs? Any concessions for learning disabilities – from 1-on-1 teaching, to extra classes, to audio-visual learning techniques – are not signs of weakness. On the contrary, they signal the strength it takes to continue in this world despite circumstances.

To demand inclusion is to say, "You cannot universalise education in a manner that excludes us. We are here and our education matters. We will have it and we will not be shamed into having it your way." To defy, to be different is a mark of courage.

So when PWDs ask for concessions, they tell the world, "We have not given up. We will not be left in the margins."

♦♦♦

Alas, this is all in retrospect. At the time, a scribe was veto-ed.

Scribe or no scribe, Krishanv was struggling to learn on a daily basis. And by the 9th grade we had had enough. The curriculum had increased in volume. No amount of after-school classes helped. The scene just ended up being a clone of school – a room of 60 where 55 stopped paying attention to the teacher because the teacher stopped paying attention to them.

There was too much to catch up to. The discrepancy between his oral and written answering began to widen. All his free time became absorbed in learning and relearning and rote-learning. He had no space to be social, no time for play. His spirits began to sink.

We couldn't stretch the band any further. His formative years were rolling by and nothing at school was working. We realised that it was time to show some true courage. To be truly defiant of an exclusionary system. If schools couldn't find the right space and expertise in which to educate our son, we'd do it our way. And so it was settled: Kitu would be homeschooled.

Chapter Ten

Did He Went from School?

Imagine everyone you know is on a ship. You have to get from shore A to shore B and *all* those who are fortunate to make the journey are on this ship. Your forefathers and some privileged foremothers made the journey too, of course on a more rudimentary boat. You've been promised it's the safest way to make the journey, tried and tested and approved by time.

You don't particularly like this ship. It moves quickly and the captain doesn't speak your language. The food is terrible too. Everyone else seems to be having a good enough time but you're bored and seasick and you have no idea where the vessel is headed.

You crane your neck over the side and look out into the sea. Some fools have decided to make the journey by rowboat. It would be a different matter if there was no place on your ship but there's plenty of room, and yet these morons have chosen to risk it on their own. Blithering idiots!

You wave at them and they wave back and you can't help but notice that unlike your's, their smiles aren't forced.

On the one hand, the ship is huge. It looks sturdier, safer than the rowboat. And literally everyone you know is on it. Everyone. There's just a couple on the rowboat but thousands on this ship. Surely, not all these people would have picked the wrong vessel. Security in numbers, right? Besides, they'd call you a fool for abandoning the ship so close to shore B.

On the other hand, the rowboat's doing just fine without size. It's all caught up with the ship and scheduled to reach shore B when you will. Everyone knows everyone else and someone is playing the bouzouki. And you're on a ship with a hundred people who couldn't care about you any more than the next stranger. Plus, they make subpar food.

Oh but the ship has worked for nearly everybody! Surely you could give it some more time? Sure, the first 4, 5, 6 years didn't workout. Maybe you just have to push a little – try harder, make more friends, learn the captain's language sooner. How hard can it be? If this ship worked just fine for a thousand before you, there's no reason it isn't perfect for you too, right?

Wrong. It's been 11 years and you've had enough. Your head is spinning and everything is grey. You cannot help but feel sick up so high above the water. You're done trying and you've made up your mind. You're going to get away from this sickening ship, from its distant people, and from the captain who won't try to understand you. You want good food. To the rowboat it is!

There's just one question: How will you get off the ship?

♦♦♦

The Ultimate Foolproof Watertight Guide to Throwing Your Child off a Ship

Step 1: Determine If This is the Best Option for Them

Start with talking to people you know who have also thrown their children off ships. While deciding what to do with Krishnav, we contacted several parents of homeschooled children and inundated them with all the questions we had.

- What about exams? You speak to the authority for your selected certification board and let them know you're homeschooling. They will send your child the same examinations that a school-going student would get.
- Is getting into college an issue? Nope. Same board exams, same cut offs.
- Does it impair classroom-learning later on? Can't say. Depends on your kid's personal studying preferences. And for all you know, they might never be in a classroom situation again.
- How do they make friends? They'll be doing a lot more than just studying at home. Peers are not difficult to come by.

We were convinced that homeschooling was right for Kitu because the parents we spoke to were more than satisfied with their children's progress. They claimed that their children had more agency over how they learned, which meant that studying seemed less like a burden. Moreover, they had more free time to do things they loved like play sports at their own time or take extra courses in things like AI and entrepreneurship.

We did wonder how we'd manage putting in the effort required to teach Kitu on our own. Himanshu was out 15 days a month and I had all the responsibilities of a working mother. To delegate the role of 'teacher' to us on top of all this seemed like the block that would topple the Jenga tower.

Thankfully, we found out that specialised tutions were in fact available. Classrooms with less than 8 students, where Krishnav would have the security of a professional teacher without the restrictions of an institution. We would have the assurance that he was getting specialised attention without the task of having to do it ourselves.

But don't just take it from us. Get as many testimonies as you can. There are several online sources for such discussions too. Find people who have been in your position and talk to them about your decision. Once you have an aggregate understanding of what you're in for, only then take a call.

By the end of this process, you should be convinced that your decision to homeschool is the right decision for your child. If it isn't, abandon the mission. Let them stay on the boat for a while longer – either till they're ready to revisit the question or for the rest of their education.

Step 2: Do the Paperwork

You can't throw someone off the ship without getting the required clearances, of course. The captain needs to be informed and such and such. It takes so. much. time. But it's imperative that you have all the clearances you need, otherwise the last minute running around takes twice the effort and nine times the stress.

We took an appointment with the principle of Krishnav's school to inform her of our decision. Thankfully, she was more than understanding. So obtaining his school-leaving certificate was the easiest of the lot. What required more effort was the process to switch boards.

Till this point, Krishnav was studying under ICSE and we'd decided to shift to SSC, the Maharashtra state board. SSC has a reputation for being lowly, meant only for students who are either slow or Marathi-speaking poor or both. It is looked down upon by the elite who can afford to send their children to English-medium private schools where ICSE and IBDP dominate.

Initially, we were also perpetrators of this baseless prejudice. One can imagine our pleasant surprise when we conducted our due diligence and perused the SSC curriculum.

We found SSC to certainly be easier than ICSE. Previously, we had equated this ease with a lower level of educational rigour, but we were grossly mistaken. SSC's ease is not a sign of its inadequacy but its strength: Teaching a child just enough of everything they need to know before deciding their specialisation for college. No more.

Every topic covered in ICSE is covered in SSC, thus it cannot be argued that it isn't a well-rounded curriculum. The difference is that ICSE tackles each subject in much detail and SSC doesn't. That is exactly its advantage.

Do you remember the first 20 elements in the Periodic Table? Could you draw and name every major Indian river on a map? Can you recall all the types of grasses in Australia?[30] Of course not! Because which middle-school child needs to know these things?

That's why specialisation exists at the undergrad level! Boards that boast a robust curriculum are usually just cramming more and more information for younger and younger children, much more than they can sustainably absorb. That's like watching your bucket overflow and then boasting about not shutting the tap.

Thus, we took Krishnav out of the rat race. Along with the school-leaving certificate, we required a No Objection Certificate and the UDISE number from

---

[30] All real questions, not joking. Your 11-14 year-old is expected to know these things. Go take a look at their textbook. Ashni recalls not understanding a thing in ISC mathematics. Three years later, she's taking an online course from MIT and the syllabus is the same. Imagine! Our 16 year-olds are rote learning things that even MIT undergrads are not expected to know before coming to the classroom!

the school to submit to the SSC certification board to officiate the switch[31]. Moreover, (after barely scraping by in French) we requested that Kitu be exempt from having to learn a new language as a concession. For this, his dyslexia certificate from the local government-attested Learning Disability Clinic came in handy.

Krishnav started homeschooling in the 9th grade but we wanted to keep this structure till he passed his 12th board exams. While this was feasible for most theory-centric subjects, we had to enroll Krishnav in highschool for the sake of practical exams. Since physics, chemistry, and biology practical assessments cannot be conducted at home, he was required to be affiliated with a formal institution[32].

We found a local college and explained the situation to them. Sadly, there is no clear legal precedent for homeschooling when an institution that is not under the Government has an attendance requirement.

Be under no illusions, red tape is real. There are few offices that handle such matters and not all applications happen online. You will have to travel, spend days meeting

---

[31] This, of course, is specific to SSC. Thus, we had to deliver the certifications to the state government's education department office. If your child is studying under another board – CBSE, IGCSE, ICSE, IBDP, ISC, or your state curriculum – there will of course be variations in what paperwork you are required to submit as well as where and how to submit them. Look for this information online or by a phone call to the relevant centre.

[32] This may not be the case for students pursuing the humanities or commerce streams.

with the relevant people to get certain confirmations. But to be honest, it's the only tough part of the process. The price of admission, literally.

Step 3: Help Your Child Row to Shore

Be in touch with their teachers. Encourage good use of the newfound free time. Be involved.

This is a crucial and possibly difficult transition. You want to be there for your child every step of the way.

Step 4: Be Prepared to Bring Them Back Aboard.

It has worked for most since it is only intuitive that more personal attention and studying tools only improves learning.

But on the off-chance that it doesn't suit your child – one reason could be because you can't devote the time to teaching and can't find a tutor – mentally prepare yourself for a gap year. It's not likely but if it occurs, you don't want to create an attitude of despair around the decision.

If homeschooling doesn't work out and your child has to return to school, they may begin to feel guilty, as if it's their fault for having not been able to make it through this journey. For the benefit of your child's morale, be mentally prepared for the failure of this experiment.

Step 5: Relax. You Now Know That Rowboats Are Safe. Go Get Some Sleep

♦♦♦

The results? SSC's simplified curriculum proved ideal for Krishnav. Now that he was not expected to simply rote learn gigabytes of information, he could actually take the time to understand the concepts he was being taught. The reduced stress also allowed him to focus and reproduce the learned material better. Now that the reasons for his resistance were taken away, he could begin to *learn* and not just *study*.

And viola! After two years of homeschooling, Krishnav passed his 10th grade boards with a stunning 78%! His spirits were high as ever, and our family cried tears of disbelieving joy.

Better yet, he has a lot more free time. He didn't need to mandatorily spend 7 hours in a classroom if he only needed 4 to learn what he had to for the day! All that extra time was channelled into his extracurricular activities, on all the things he never had the time to pursue because of a burdensome curriculum. He began robotics classes. His team ranked 4th all over the country in the World Robotics Championship. The same kid who couldn't stand two minutes in the classroom without drifting off now he spent hours working relentlessly on a single project!

Later, under the guidance of a family friend and software engineer, Krishnav started developing websites. He's now fluent in multiple computer languages, surprising his mentor with his skill and passion. And again, the student who couldn't spell 4-letter words now writes pages and pages of functional code!

What's more, he recently founded his own rental platform through an entrepreneurship workshop for adolescents and pitched it to a panel of reputable businesswomen. For this, he won first place at ISME's *Think Young Entrepreneurs* competition. It's wonderful what children can do when they have the time to be creative!

To answer the big one: No, he's not lonely at all. He doesn't miss school, and is still in touch with some of his classmates. What's more, he met most of his now closest friends after we began homeschooling. He was surrounded by wonderful children at tuitions and other extracurricular classes like squash and theatre. Not to mention all the children who live in our vicinity. Every evening in our locality, girls and boys of 11 to 18 y-o-a gather in one parking ground or another to play football or cricket, ride hoverboards or bicycles, or chase each other around with Nerf guns. There is nothing in the world that will convince Krishnav to give up the slot in his day dedicated to this revelry.

There is no way to overstate the positive impact homeschooling had on our lives. Krishnav's tutors are an unimaginably wholesome duo. They were the most accommodating of tutors who never relented till Kitu'd learnt his work as thoroughly as any other student. More importantly, they knew how to interweave Krishnav's special learning needs with their expectations. Methodology and pace were suited as per his requirements. Their compassion and love for their students, coupled with their passion for their job meant the pair was a formula made for success. They had faith in his abilities and children can sense that. I think Krishnav's improved scores came more out of the pleasure of learning than the pressure of scoring.

How did the rest of us fare, you ask? For starters, I realised my child was a *part* of my life, not my whole life.

All this allowed me to create an identity for myself beyond that of a mother. Able to give time and mental energy to my work, I found my calling and passion aside from my duties. None of this would've been possible at a regular school. I am so glad we made this decision, and I would've made it sooner if I'd known.

Of course, it hasn't been a level road. Every instance has tested my strength. But it has been worth it, for we have been surprised by our own resilience. Through every ebb and flow, we've learnt and grown. Every bump we met with courage, and upon emerging stronger we knew our faith was not in vain.

"What does Krishnav do?" I remember being asked by a doctor, himself diagnosed with ADD. "High-school. He's been struggling but he works hard and makes it through most things." "Let me tell you something about us. When we are interested in something, we pursue it with all our heart. What's his interest?"

"Computer science."

"Then he will do wonders in computer science. Trust me, he's going to be fine."

There you have it, from the horse's mouth. Our children are going to be fine.

Hope is an intoxicant. Exhilarating and adventurous.

Keep the faith. Good times are just around the corner.

Et Tu?
Others Speak

सावधानी हटी, दुर्घटना घटी // **Sāvdhānī Haṭī, Durghaṭnā Ghaṭī**

It didn't take long after Jarul Thakur was born before she had established herself as a mischievous one.

Once, at about 3 y-o-a, while making rounds of the house looking for something to fidget with, she found an ideal target. On a Shimla morning like any other, her father sat engrossed in his reading with a cup of *chai* and his cellphone on a table by his side. "This was the time of those big Nokia phones," recalls her mother, a teacher herself, "And Jarul couldn't sit still..."

Tip-tapping to the table, Jarul rushed to the object of mischief, picked up her father's phone and dunked it into his cup of *chai*! By the time he realised what had happened, the little trouble-maker had scurried off, looking for the next play thing.

"मैंने नहीं किया! (*Mené nahī.n kīyā!*) I didn't do it!" she laughed. No wonder Mrs. Thakur had lovingly named her 'सावधानी हटी, दुर्घटना घटी (*Sāvdhānī Haṭī, Durghaṭnā Ghaṭī*)'[33]!

---

[33] Hindi for 'look away for a moment, and the crisis has occurred'.

Another time, Mrs. Thakur came home from work to find all the house plants shining in the sun. Perplexed, she went up to examine what magic had found its way into her home. As she got closer, she found that dozens of leaves had been punctured through with all-pins!

Sigh. Jarul was promptly summoned and without hesitation she said, "But now the monkeys won't try to eat the plants!"

Way to problem-solve! You have to admit, no classroom teaches such creativity.

So it's little surprise that this out-of-the-box thinker didn't fare well within the lines that mainstream education tried to draw around her. By the time she reached the 2nd Grade, it was obvious to her mother that Jarul's academic performance indicated something more fundamental. Her spellings were often jumbled and her memory was wanting. "While reading long paragraphs, she would have trouble with even simple words," testifies Mrs. Thakur, "and after she'd read a word, she might forget it instantly, having to re-learn it if it cropped up again in the next line.

"So I decided to go to the school counsellor." At the time, the counsellor didn't recommend any tests. He believed nothing was amiss, despite the evidence Jarul's mother had brought along with her. And so 2nd Grade went by and 3rd Grade trudged behind. It was only later that Jarul's performance at school began demanding graver attention.

With only 40s and 50s out of a 100 marks under her belt, Jarul became the object of her class teacher's ridicule. "The teacher would throw her notebook across the room, berating her before the whole class for her handwriting."

> *You're good for nothing!*
> *You need treatment!*
>
> अपनी माँ से पढ़ के आ! *(Apnī Mā sé padh ké ā!) Go, get your mother to teach you!*

In one of India's oldest schools and one of Shimla's best convents, Jarul was mocked by the very professionals tasked with nurturing her. Every day, she faced caustic comments – if not from the teachers then from the teacher's pets. How are our children to maintain any self-confidence, when all around them figures of authority crush spirits like dry leaves under their heels?

"I didn't know how bad it was at first," says Mrs. Thakur. Now in the 4th Grade, this lil one was the school's Sports Captain. A star athlete at every game she picked up, there was no doubt she was more than deserving of her badge.

Imagine the disappointment when she was prohibited from attending a single interschool sports competition! Citing her low grades as an excuse, her teachers made her wait back in the classroom and work on her studies while her teammates went off to do what they loved. For no benefit, they held her back from developing her strengths, from honing her talents. So much for holistic excellence.

"And then this one time, she'd been looking low for days. I asked her if something had happened, and she burst out crying..."

Jarul had been taken to the Principal's office over some inflamed accusation. The Principal, bellowed over the 10 y-o child, making full use of absolute, unaccountable power. All of a sudden, mid-bellow, he slapped his hands beneath the table that separated him from Jarul and flipped it into the air.

Up. Twirl. Come crashing down.

"I didn't tell you because I didn't want to get into trouble," she managed between teary hiccups, "If you go complain, the teachers will only make things more difficult for me..." Unknown to Jarul, Mrs. Thakur was at school the next day. A teacher herself, she gave the Principal his due, reminding him of his place of responsibility. "If I'm alright with my child's performance, who are your teachers to attack her self-esteem for it?"

Boiling point. It was time to move to a school with a conscience. Jarul's parents found another institution in Shimla, this one more to their liking. The Founder soon became a cornerstone of all the support and consideration that Jarul received. Even before her diagnosis – which only came a few months after she enrolled – he had shown absolute empathy for her sensitivities. He'd personally instructed all her teachers, ensuring they neither made her question her self-worth nor pressured her to learn the way her peers did.

"He was her pillar," says Mrs. Thakur. Over the next 4 years, the Founder and other teachers found a way to make mainstream education deliver for Jarul. A sharp contrast from her previous classrooms, her new environment was one of consideration and understanding. With genuine concern and a sense of duty towards their jobs, they gave this little one the additional attention she needed to keep up with her class. There's nothing caregivers can't achieve when armed with empathy for their children. Soon Jarul's scores began to improve and her self-confidence was restored.

But what off her hyperactivity? Mrs. Thakur still had this one Sysiphisian task at hand.

A malady came forth organically and surely. Recognising the creativity brimming from this little one, Mrs. Thakur filled up Jarul's spare time with doodling and music. Like a shoot pushing out through the surface of the earth, all that energy within her took form. As strokes on paper or riding on airwaves, Jarul's ability to focus grew firmer and firmer.

Over the years, these management techniques have helped Jarul cope sustainably with mainstream education. With no formal special educators / remedial therapists and by the sheer will of involved parents and teachers, today this mischief-maker copes in a system that wasn't designed for learners like her. Best of all, she won't compromise her creativity for it.

Today, to meet Jarul is to be in awe of her maturity, her every talent, and her spirit. "खुराफाती बच्ची (*khurāfātī bachchī*)," laughs her mother, "ग़दर मचाती है! (*Gadar machātī hai!*)"[34]

◆◆◆

Master of Her Trade

Aditi Gandhi's journey began when a teacher noticed that the 4 year-old's impatience to complete her work was beginning to distract the class. The teacher suspected there was something more to Aditi's hyperactivity than indiscipline. Learning of these concerns, radiologists Dr. and Dr. Gandhi decided to formally test it. They wished to weed out the other possible hindrances to her learning before believing she had ADHD.

Aditi underwent an IQ test as well as a BERA scan to ensure her auditory senses were not the problem. Both tests came back with satisfactory results. The doctors concluded that Aditi probably had ADHD.

Probably. Nothing could be said for certain, so the conclusion was ignored. There seemed no need for further diagnosis until her grades began to fall drastically by the time she was fourteen. In the seventh grade, Aditi was formally tested and diagnosed positive for Dyslexia, Dysgraphia, and Dyscalculia. The Gandhis were devastated. This was difficult to accept.

---

[34] Hindi for 'Mischievous girl! She cannot be contained!'

For Aditi, secondary school was emotionally draining since she was ostracised from her peer group. Loneliness is common among ADHD and Dyslexic students, as school faculty and students are not trained to sympathise with learning disabilities. Aditi began to eat her sadness. Finding solace in food, she became unhealthier. An unfit body can't help a struggling mind, and learning further became a task.

Word problems posed a great challenge. Comprehending long paragraphs at a stretch was an uphill battle. Again, her mother came to her rescue! Dr. Gandhi placed a ruler below the line being read, making it easier for Aditi not to jump sentences. Genius!

Despite all the hurdles – the LD, the ostracism, the weight gain – Aditi scored a 72% in her 10th boards. Thankfully, she was among the lucky few in this country who was able to avail concessions for a writer by her side.

Onward to her undergraduate studies, Aditi faced resistance from ignorant bystanders who claimed the sciences would be too challenging for her. But this young fighter could not be pressured into giving up her dreams just because someone else didn't have faith in them. She went on to acquire a BASLP degree in Audiology and Speech.

Now pursuing her Masters in the same, Aditi is the perfect mentor for the special-needs children who seek her help. She sympathises with their predicament and knows the ins and outs of their experiences of being "different" in society. She uses the knowledge from her own experiences to modify established practices to suit children with LDs. She is passionate about her work, which defies any inhibitions that a disability could possibly impose.

Aditi is a beacon of hope to students with disabilities who know the brunt of social pressures to follow convention. She has traversed labels and stigma, insensitivity and injustice. For every time words have tried to push her down, she's risen stronger. Today, she has blossomed into a fine young woman who speaks her grit and never says die.

♦♦♦

देर आये, दुरुस्त आये // Dér Āyé, Durust Āyé

During his 3rd year doing MBBS at Father Muller Medical College, Dr. Sandeep P. T. was required to take a clinical posting in Psychiatry. Perusing the reading material, he became especially interested in the checklist to diagnose ADHD:

- Inability to concentrate for extended periods of time.
- Inability to sit still without fidgeting.
- Starting new tasks before completing current ones…

It was like looking in a mirror. "I could identify with almost each and every one," he says.

In all his school years, Sandeep had sensed something was amiss. He could never focus in a classroom and got 0s in his tests. "My best subject was Biology," he recalls, "I regularly got Cs and Ds in it! Haha!" Comparing himself to his peers, he'd ask why he was consistently lacking. But of course, there was no fault in his efforts, so there was no answer to be found within.

ADD is just attention deficiency, no hyperactivity. It has similar implications on learning but without the overt displays of restlessness. "I spoke to my HOD at college. I told him about how I could relate to what I had read in my textbook. He confirmed, I had ADD. Now everything made sense."

Immediately, Sandeep called up his mother and told her of this development. "I know," she said, to his surprise, "We'd taken you to a doctor when you were young. He'd said the same thing and prescribed some meds for you but we didn't really think much of it." Sandeep's spirits sank. If only he'd been informed when he was younger, there was much that could've been done to support him through his schooling years.

But *khair*. देर आये, दुरुस्त आये (*dér āyé, durust āyé*) – better late than never. He'd missed the Early Intervention deadline but thank god "Late Intervention" is an open invite. Sandeep began to train his brain to focus better on important tasks, to retain information. He began religiously listing and organizing, making up for what he lost to his disorder with mammoth uphill effort. "And I began helping my friends self-diagnose too!" he laughs,

"You'd be surprised how many people don't know they have learning disabilities."

While disabilities among resourceful, privileged folks is one thing, disabilities among the lowest strata is a whole other ballgame. Sandeep worked towards healthcare in Kalahandi's tribal locales for 2 years. Operating closely with Odisha's public school teachers, he'd often hear the same rhetoric around *adivasi* students' performances –

> *They are all weak!*
> *Each dumber than the next!*
> *Useless, the whole lot of them!*

But what he saw himself was not a backward group whose young were too slow to learn. No. What he found instead was a systemically disenfranchised population, many of whom were undiagnosed special-needs children. And when ADHD children with privilege face unbelievable obstacles, we can assume that the path for marginalised communities is paved with thorns.

"When you're rich, you have privilege. If you're poor but bright, everyone wants to help you." he laments, "Who helps the rest? What about the lowest income bracket with disabilities?"

There are many such marginalised groups in India whose children have known only poverty all their lives. With the prevalent levels of malnutrition, the lack of exposure to mainstream society, and the pressures of a low-income household, how can you expect these children to flourish in a mainstream classroom?

I wonder what is in store for India's ignored children. I guess that's our community's next challenge – The first was waking up to learning disabilities as worthy of empathy and support. Now it is to make education work for all children as a right rather than a privilege. To make learning effective beyond differences in abilities, beyond differences in geography, beyond the hierarchies of privilege.

Expert-Speak

Rukshan Vakil
M. A. Dip SLD-Dyslexia (UK), AMCollT (London)
Clinical Psychologist and Remedial Educator;
Associate – College of Teaching (London)
RCI Reg. No.: AO2247

I am a Clinical Psychologist and Remedial Educator, practicing since 1990. I have worked with a varied age demographic. My focused niche is children and teenagers with Specific Learning Disorders (SLDs), Attention Deficit Disorders (ADDs), and those with Special Needs. Besides private consultation, I am associated with schools that have an inclusive education policy, where I conduct assessments, diagnoses, and awareness and remedial programmes.

The Basics

ADDs and SLDs range from 'mild' to 'severe'. Often, mild cases are not detected or diagnosed. We all probably know a dozen adults who battle the obstacles of these disorders on a daily basis, never understanding why they must work a little harder each day than the average person.

Students with ADDs have it the worst at schools. With closed spaces and disciplinary requirements, they are unable to sit still. They require structured breaks, or else may feel constricted and restless. This of course impacts their concentration towards their academics and their holistic mental well-being.

Students with SLDs face difficulties with basic academic curricula – reading, writing, and arithmetic. They are expected to adhere to the literacy requirements of education systems that often stifle their creativity and uniqueness as they advance through to higher grades.

Standardized Tests

There is no standard way of having a human mind, and no standard way of being a child. Experienced Psychologists and Educators can detect and diagnose SLD / ADD with or without standardized tests through informal and curriculum based achievement tests, case history and analysis of the child's work.

However, standardized tests have become a necessity to obtain necessary accommodations and provisions at the Secondary and Higher Secondary level, especially with the profusion of schools in Mumbai following international boards of education.

It is important to remember that cultural differences impact how different communities' students respond to tests. And those who design these tests may not always be from the same culture as the student giving the test. Most standardized tests are Western and have not been adjusted specifically for Indian students. They however, can and are used with children, who have an English-speaking home and school background.

Diagnosis and Labeling

Diagnosis is important to work with the specific areas of difficulty and plan remedial programmes. However, being labelled can have both advantages and hazardous effects to a student's self-esteem.

On the one hand, it can provide a sense of ease. Upon understanding that they have a learning disability and are not simply "dumb" or "stupid", the students breathes a sigh of relief, letting go of the stress that their low performance is their fault. They now have the confidence that the people around them too will understand and will cease to blame the student themselves. They are more assured that they will be guided on the path to improved learning.

On the other hand, students are known to detest being labelled as 'Resource Room Kids'. It invites bullying from other students, which leads to isolation. This may cause a reluctance to go to school or participate in academics. It may also cause psychosomatic aches and pains.

Remedial Work

Disorders are not diseases, hence there is no cure. However, there are many structured programmes that can help overcome symptoms and ease daily functioning.

Early Intervention in the form of speech therapy, sensory integration or remedial work has historically proven successful for many. There is a positive correlation between the immediacy of intervention and the improvement in students' performances i.e. getting help when in primary school is better than starting in secondary school.

Just like standardized tests, remedial programmes are not one-size-fits-all. Early remedial work focuses on the basics of phonics, reading, writing, and arithmetic as well as perceptual and visual-motor skills. In later years, the emphasis shifts to tutorial-based therapy to improve memory, concentration, comprehension, and creative writing. The frequency and duration of remedial work varies, but generally children continue till high-school. Results are not immediately evident and the tendency to discontinue midway is common. Consistency and persistence are important to reap the full benefits.

Masarrat Khan

Structured Literacy Dyslexia Specialist (USA)
Certified Academic Language Therapist (USA)
Chief Executive Officer – Maharashtra Dyslexia Association (MDA)
Registered Rehabilitation Psychologist – Rehabilitation Council of India

With three decades of experience in the field, I am responsible for the programmes for psychologists and special educators with the Maharashtra Dyslexia Association (MDA). I am also the course-coordinator for the Dyslexia Therapist Training Programme – the first of its kind in India.

Are ADDs and Dyslexia Similar?

They are independent of one another but can co-exist as well.

Many Dyslexic students are misdiagnosed with ADDs due to their restlessness or inattentiveness in class. This restlessness, though may not come from a disorder but from their inability to keep pace with the class.

Many ADD students are also misdiagnosed with SLDs. Students with ADDs may dislike writing because it requires focus and attention, which is difficult for them. They may be simply impulsive and impatient, which manifests as shabby notebooks and illegible writing mistaken as signs of an SLD.

At What Age is Diagnosis Possible / Appropriate?

As early as 5 years-old, when formal education begins. But this stage may come later for some children, which is simply a matter of personal development and doesn't imply a worse case of the disorder.

What to Do If Standardised Tests Are Not Always Appropriate for Indian Students?

The National Brain Research Centre's Dyslexia Assessment for Languages of India (DALI) is now available in English, Hindi, Marathi, Kannada, and Tamil.

More information about these is available online.

Are Remedials Helpful?

Yes, it is the only way to help a student with SLDs / ADDs. As long as the methods are grounded in empirical science, of course.

For Dyslexia, it is highly recommended to use remedial methods based on the Orton-Gillingham guidelines. I myself have worked with individuals of ages 4 to 41 years, and thus can attest that such methods are beneficial even for adults.

What's the Indian Scene Like?

Indians are definitely under-diagnosed, since social awareness about and acceptance of SLDs is dismal. Fortunately, the discussion is opening up, and I personally know of students with SLDs in every field – from medicine, law, and engineering to architecture, software, and hospitality.

MDA was closely involved in the making of *Taare Zameen Par*. The film was a breakthrough in terms of bringing the Indian public to terms with the reality of the existence of SLDs. All you have to do today is name the movie and almost everyone familiar with Bollywood immediately thinks, "Dyslexia!"

In the decades prior to the film's release, it would've been nearly impossible that the average Indian would be able to name a single SLD. Unfortunately, just a movie is not enough to entirely dissolve a social stigma, and India students remain underdiagnosed, even if at a reduced rate.

Further, those who do have the privilege of a diagnosis often do not get the required assistance at home or school. Rather, all they get is the stigma attached to the label. Furthermore, successful professionals with SLDs often do not wish to talk about their journeys for the fear of being misunderstood or marginalised, either at the workplace or society in general.

The globe and especially India still has a long way to go in making education a safe and inclusive space for all kinds of learners. The good news is that people like you, the Acharyas, and organisations like MDA won't stop till we're there!

Epilogue

Our dear protagonist Krishnav has penned the following section. To maintain the spirit of this book, we've left it as is with not a comma edited. Enjoy!

Epilogue of Kitu's adventure

My adventure has been very amazing lately I love to think that whenever I am in pain or I am unwell for some reason I think that I have superpowers and trust at the age of 17 I still think about it, and everytime I think about these things I say only one thing my brain is my superpower.I like to take my Dyslexia also as a superpower and make it my strength not my weakness.I am going to be honest with you guys the journey I have been in with my brain and me being a Dyslexiac I love it I am thinking a thousand things while I am doing one thing I get a lot headaches but I got to know how to control some and maybe as I grow up and mature I will be able to take all the pain away. So please read my book it's written not to make me famous but more importantly to help a mother with a Disleyic,hyper,unmature child to grow up! My aim is I want this book to reach high writers and make this book revolutionary so whenever a mother has a problem she can tell her son by reading this book that how to behave and mature properly.

I am just going to say this last thing, "I Think the way you say it and make a child understand it through a different approach matters".Thankyou very much

Printed in Great Britain
by Amazon